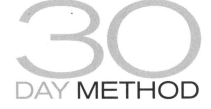

TRACY ANDERSON'S
30
DAY METHOD

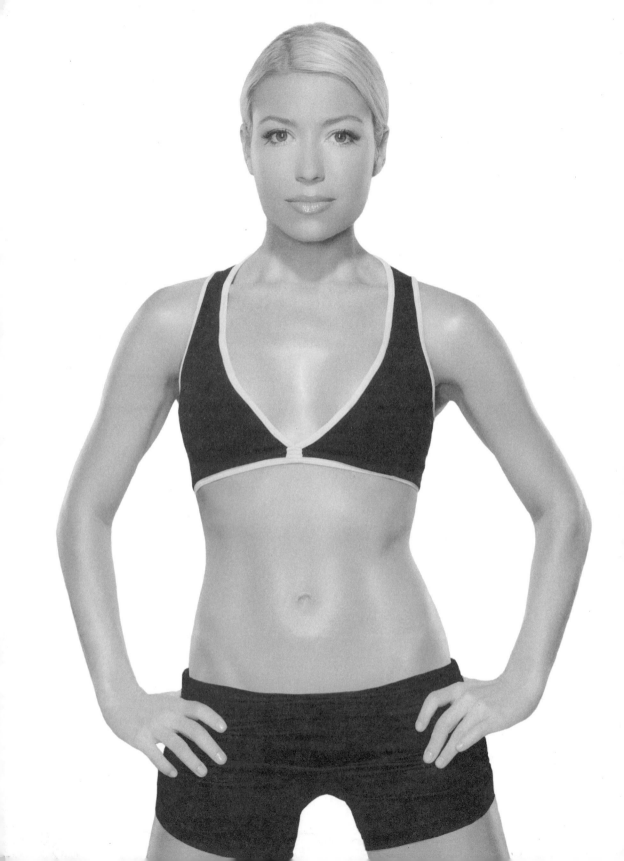

TRACY ANDERSON'S
30
DAY METHOD

THE WEIGHT-LOSS KICK-START THAT MAKES PERFECTION POSSIBLE

Tracy Anderson

with a Foreword by Gwyneth Paltrow

GRAND CENTRAL
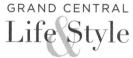
Life & Style
NEW YORK · BOSTON

Book and DVD copyright © 2010 by T.A. Studios LLC

Grand Central Life & Style
Hachette Book Group
1290 Avenue of the Americas
New York, NY 10104

www.HachetteBookGroup.com

Grand Central Life & Style is an imprint of Grand Central Publishing.
The Grand Central Life & Style name and logo are trademarks of Hachette Book Group, Inc.

The Hachette Speakers Bureau provides a wide range of authors for speaking events. To find out more, go to www.hachettespeakersbureau.com or call (866) 376-6591.

The publisher is not responsible for websites (or their content) that are not owned by the publisher.

Printed in the United States of America

Originally published in hardcover by Grand Central Life & Style.

First Trade Edition: May 2012
10 9 8 7 6 5 4 3 2

The Library of Congress has cataloged the hardcover edition as follows:

Anderson, Tracy.
  Tracy Anderson's 30-day method : the weight-loss kick-start that makes perfection possible / Tracy Anderson.—1st ed.
    p. cm.
  Includes index.
  ISBN 978-0-446-56204-1
  1. Reducing exercises. 2. Weight loss. 3. Exercise for women. I. Title. II. Title: Tracy Anderson's thirty-day method.
  RA781.6.A545 2010
  613.2.'5—dc22

                                        2010007884

ISBN 978-0-446-56205-8 (pbk.)

Book Design by Renato Stanisic

To my Mother, Diana Jean Blythe Ephlin
I am one of the lucky ones. I am the daughter of a perfect mother. She has always had
fairy dust around her from the time I was born.

*   *   *

To my Father, Robert Scott Richardson
Sometimes our life's greatest challenges can be gifts. My father is inventive and
brilliant but was vested in many ideas. So I rebelled by staying focused on one thing. So
now I have a fitness Method.

*   *   *

To Nanny and Poppa
When you are a creative person to be successful I believe you need a sense of solid. They
instilled my sense of solid.

*   *   *

To my Partner, Gwyneth Paltrow
Celebrity culture is an interesting paradigm. We all have those that inspire us from
afar but we never really know the person behind the inspiration. Gwyneth is inspiration
and magic from every dimension. She is truly my mentor in life.

*   *   *

To my Son, Sam Anderson
He is my Beacon. My home.

Contents

Foreword

I first met Tracy Anderson in 2006 on a busy afternoon in New York City. I had heard about her from a mutual friend who had raved that Tracy had changed her body and her life, and I was curious to see what lay in store. Never could I have imagined when she opened the door, tiny and blonde and smiling, how much of an impact she would have, not only on my physical body, but also on the road that lay ahead. She promptly stripped me down and sized me up. I was still a good 15 pounds over the weight I like to be after having my second child, my boy, and no matter what I did I could not shift the weight, let alone tighten up. A devotee of yoga and Pilates for years, I had long ago given up on changing my shape or having a body I would have asked for. I was always skinny on top and on the bottom, well, not so much. "Hmm" I heard her tut while she was measuring my upper outer thigh, commonly known to us ladies as saddlebags. "These have got to go." She said that I would be easy to change, that it would take some hard work but in time it would happen. I was dubious. I had always been disciplined in my workouts and had never had real results: What did she know that no one else did?

The answer was made clear that day and in the coming months. Tracy's ingenious and unique method completely changed my body, so much so that it made headlines. Not only did she get me out of my maternity jeans, she got me into clothes I wouldn't have worn ten years earlier. And along with the physical change came an incredible empowerment. The results were proportionate to the effort put in; never had I experienced that before. I felt strong and vital. I felt capable of anything.

The road there was tough, never had I felt so sore. The muscular structure work was difficult as hell but the dance aerobics was worse; I never realized how truly uncoordinated I was until I tried to dance. I was so gangly that at first my "dance cardio" had to consist of stepping from one side to the other and bouncing on a mini trampoline. But my body changed quickly; after doing the famous "first 10 days" of the program, I had lost 14 inches. With much practice and occasional humiliation, I became a dancer—not a good one, mind you, but good enough to do 45 minutes of rigorous aerobics, meaning I don't have to count calories to keep the weight off. And for someone who loves to cook and eat as much as I do, it means freedom. As long as I stick to Tracy's program, I can truly enjoy my life.

In the ensuing years, through life's incredible ups and downs, Tracy and I have become like family. She is constantly amazing me, not only with her insanely creative, ever-evolving fitness systems, but also with her work ethic, her beautifully generous heart, and her dedication to changing women everywhere. With this book, Tracy shares all of her secrets and gives us the opportunity to take our lives, bodies and health to the next level, whatever that may be.

Gwyneth Paltrow
April 2010

PART ONE

YOU ARE HOW YOU MOVE

1

Introduction

Welcome to the Tracy Anderson Method

If you picked up this book, even if you're just flipping through it at the bookstore, it's because you wonder if it's really possible to reinvent the shape you're in. If you bought this book and brought it home, it's because you're ready to make your dreams real.

Everybody wants to be in better shape. But have you ever considered that your body could really be problem-area-free, with toned, shapely arms, the perfect butt, and the legs of a dancer? My clients know that their genetic background won't keep them from looking gorgeous. That women who have had one, two, even three children can still look forward to buying a bathing suit. That getting older can mean getting stronger and sexier. Have you ever looked at a celebrity magazine and thought: *I could never look like that*? You can. You absolutely can. With the right workout program, you can be healthy, strong, fit, feminine, and sexy—and still be able to eat real food.

Imagine how amazing it would feel to have a physique that allowed you to move with grace, energy levels that let you keep moving all day, and a body that felt lean and defined. This book is your invitation into a world where food is not a struggle. Where physical fitness is a way of life, not an unreachable dream. Where your clothes slip on easily and everything looks great. Where your stomach is trim and flat, your arms are tight and toned, your butt and thighs look as great in jeans as they do in a bikini—all of this, and more, is achievable.

To many of you, this might sound like a fantasy. But I promise: No matter what brought you here, no matter what your current weight or what your personal story is, success is possible.

After more than a decade of working with women who, until they discovered my Tracy Anderson Method, were struggling with their weight, I can honestly say that there isn't a problem area I haven't seen. Or a dieting story that shocks me. But even after meeting and talking with hundreds and hundreds of women about their physical fitness histories, I am still moved to tears by their desire: Their desire to be desirable. Their desire to be healthy. Their desire to feel good in their clothes and sexy naked.

What moved me eleven years ago, the first time somebody sat down and cried to me about her struggles, moves me today. When I see the woman who had gastric bypass surgery but couldn't afford the full-body skin tuck after. The mother who has given birth to three beautiful children—and now has a stomach that she would like to never expose again. The executive who works out every day, obsessively, but never sees her hard work at the gym net her the success she really wants. Or the teenage girls terrified that exercise will bulk them up, so they replace sweating with starving, experimenting with eating disorders in order to stay tiny. Or those of you who have suffered through the liquid diets, the mental self-abuse, and the internal imbalance that come along with simply wanting to like what you see.

I created this program because I've been there myself. I know what it feels like to want to make a change but not have the right tools. Or to be constantly offered "solutions" that take up a lot of time and energy and money and don't really solve anything.

I created the Method because it was time for something better.

There Is a Real Solution

The work I do is rewarding because I get to watch Cinderella stories every day. I know the heartache of being overweight, of trying to make a change, and of missing the mark time and again. And I know how big a woman's smile is when she finally sees herself as the princess that she is.

I'm here to tell you that perfection really is possible. That results are really achievable. And I am the proof.

You know those girls you see with the "fast metabolisms," the kind who can eat everything they want and never gain an ounce? That is totally not me. I am not genetically blessed in the weight department. But I also don't like to deny myself the simple pleasures of delicious food. I can just look at cake and gain weight, but that doesn't mean I can imagine a life without it.

Before I developed my Method, back when I was overweight and trying to figure out how to trim down, I tried everything (you'll learn more about that in the next chapter). I was desperate. That struggle was the catalyst for the development of my Method. It opened a wound within me that I needed to heal, and helping myself and other women transform into lean, lithe goddesses became my manifesto.

Today I have more than a decade of experience transforming women's bodies into their leanest, tightest incarnations. If you commit to it, my program will free you from a lifetime of struggling with your weight, with your fitness routine, and with the knowledge that even though you work hard, you don't see the results you want.

Do you want a fit, toned body that is beautiful and full of energy? If you begin tomorrow, in just a month's time you will have completely reinvented the way your body looks and moves, boosted your self-confidence, and reset your standards for your life.

The Method Can Change Your Life—If You Let It

If you want to see real change, you can't just read about it. You have to get up and do it. You have to make a change in order to see a change. So I'm going to ask you to have a moment of truth. I'm going to ask you to commit to the three parts of my 30-Day Method: the Muscle Design Work, the Cardio Complement, and an eating plan.

Common wisdom tells you that you need to move your body and watch what you eat. But it isn't just about moving or reducing calories; it's about *how* you move and *what* kind of energy you provide for yourself.

Each part of the Method is integral to your success, and each requires your full commitment. If you commit to my 30-Day Method, I will redesign your body. If you work hard, I promise you results. Over the course of the program, you will be achieving mastery. You will feel and understand your body in a new way. That's because I'm not a trainer. I'm a choreographer, a researcher, a designer, and a teacher.

This 30-Day Method is your kick-start program, your entry into a lifestyle that will get you to your weight loss goals—and then keep you there. Listen, we all want to be slim, desirable, feminine, and sexy. None of us wants to struggle uselessly toward an unreachable goal. This is the solution that will work for the long term. Some people have resigned themselves to the misunderstanding that exercise is for health benefits alone but does not deliver weight loss results. With the 30-Day Method, you can do both: improve your health and beautify your body, successfully and sustainably.

This kick start is a boot camp that is going to shock your system and redesign your body no matter what your level of fitness or your genetic heritage. It is an intensive program that uses muscle work, cardio dance aerobics, and a menu plan to restructure your muscles, burn fat, and get you started on your way to being fit, healthy, and in better shape than you've ever dreamed.

No matter where your problems areas are, if you partner with me I will redesign your body with this 30-Day Method.

Component #1: Muscle Design Work

For the 30-Day Method Muscle Design, we go to the mats. Comprising three 10-day sequences, this portion of the program targets your smaller, secondary muscle groups, what I call the accessory muscles. Traditional workouts build the major muscle groups like your biceps, quads, and hamstrings, making them larger and adding bulk to your frame. My Method develops the smaller muscles around the bigger ones, contracting and pulling them in without creating the trauma that causes them to build bulk, so you tighten in instead of building out. This elongates, tones, and ultimately creates a smaller body structure. And by changing the moves you're doing every ten days, you ensure that your muscles stay alert and active while you tighten your skin, shape your body, burn the fat away, and consequently own the results.

Component #2: Cardio Complement

The second critical part of my plan is this high-intensity cardio dance workout. I call it the "complement" because it works in concert with your Muscle Design so that while you're giving yourself the resistance training you need to sculpt your muscles on the mat, you are also raising your heart rate in strategic intervals in order to burn excess fat at an astonishing rate. All cardio is not created equal! Some dance aerobics classes can be stop-and-go—so you never get the continuous movement needed to really burn calories. And repetitive aerobic activities, such as running or Spinning, bulk up your major muscle groups. My cardio is both continuous and varied, so you are tightening and toning while you build your endurance, burn fat, and support the hard work you're doing on the mat.

Component #3: Menu Plan

The third piece of the puzzle is my fat-loss-promoting and delicious eating plan. By putting an emphasis on foods high in nutrients and fiber, by eliminating the culprits of weight gain and bloat, you'll learn a whole new way of eating that tastes good, makes you feel great, and works with (not against!) the exercise components of the plan. As you follow this dynamic eating plan, you will kick-start your metabolism and optimize your ability to burn fat, allowing you to reach your weight loss goals in the fastest and healthiest way possible.

ONCE YOU'VE COMPLETED your 30-Day Method transformation, not only will you feel more alive because you've woken up the muscles in your body that were sleeping, but you will be free from any guilt about the food choices you make—and from having to make excuses for why your exercise routine isn't giving you the figure you want. You'll awaken and educate your system with my specific, targeted 30-Day Kick Start, and then you'll be well on your way to the body you've always wanted.

Is it really possible to reengineer my body? you may be asking. The answer is yes. No matter what your genetic background, it is absolutely possible.

2

Tracy's Story

Why I Created the Method

This system is very personal for me. It grew out of my experiences as a dancer, my struggle with my weight, my frustration with the lack of precise answers from the fitness world, and my curiosity about the human body and what it is capable of.

Why did all the trendy exercise regimens I tried seem to work at the beginning and then stop working, I started wondering. Was there a way to get off the roller coaster of weight gain and loss? Were my excuses—that I was big-boned, that this was my genetic inheritance—really excuses, or were they facts? And the biggest question of all: Was it even possible to develop a structure that I clearly wasn't naturally given? Can every woman, regardless of body type, achieve a "teeny tiny" dancer's body through exercise?

In order to fully understand my Method—and why I developed it—you have to understand where I'm coming from. I grew up in Noblesville, a very small town in Indiana, where I had a magical childhood, full of music, dancing, and creativity. My mother, who is very talented, owns a dance studio called The Dancing Place, which she opened when I was four. My mom is athletic; my dad is the opposite. He's built like Danny DeVito. So I definitely did not have a genetic step up when it came to being physically fit.

Lucky for me, my role model, my mom, always encouraged me to dance. I spent every day at her studio. She's a very gifted instructor. Most teachers just bark form and repetition, but Mom recognized the importance of presence. Instead of typical recitals, she would put on full-length ballets like *Giselle*, *Coppelia*, and *Swan Lake* because she wanted every student to understand what I later realized to be one of the most important keys to my Method: connection. It was from my mom that I learned that you have to be present and connected, and from her that I learned the difference between doing something and really *performing* it.

Those are amazing memories for me. But by the time I started thinking about college, everything had changed. My parents' marriage ended, and my mom was left with three kids and no support. She had the dance studio, but it didn't generate enough income. To help pick up the pieces, she continued teaching dance and took on two other jobs to support us. This is where I learned to have the strength to make tough choices. Like figuring out how I would go to college even though there wasn't any money for me to do so.

Things looked bleak, but I had learned from my mom how important it was to stick with it and not give up. Despite circumstances, I knew what I wanted to do.

"Mom," I said, having decided to beat the odds, no matter what it took. "I really want to go to dance school in New York."

The Freshman Forty

I got to New York with twenty dollars in my pocket, soon joined by a key to a dorm room full of cockroaches. I was over the moon. I auditioned into all the highest-level dance classes at my school. This was what I had wanted my entire life. I was thrilled, and terrified, but most of all, I was grateful. I couldn't believe the lengths my mom had gone to in order to help me get closer to my dream of being a dancer, and I was determined to show her my appreciation by being a success. Then I started gaining weight. Everything changed. I kept putting on pounds, even after my instructors started nodding their heads at me or making comments. Five pounds became ten, and the comments became more pointed.

Then it was fifteen pounds, and I would cry to Mom, who would tell me it was just the freshman fifteen. But then it became the freshman forty.

I was struggling, and I was confused. I couldn't understand why my body was becoming heavier even though I spent all day with my foot up on the barre. Dancers aren't supposed to be heavy. They aren't even supposed to be curvy. My teachers were disappointed, and I was miserable—my weight gain wasn't just making me feel bad about myself, it was ruining my shot at a career. You can imagine my five-foot-tall forty-pounds-heavier frame squeezing into a black leotard and pale pink tights. At dance school, being overweight is simply not an option.

One of my instructors actually dropped me down to a different level because of my body. It wasn't about my skill, it was about my figure. He said to me, "If Disney stays on Broadway, Ms. Anderson, you'll have plenty of work." So that was my future: I would be a teapot. That was not at all what I had pictured. I wanted to be the ingénue, not a useful piece of china.

When you go to school on a dance scholarship, they expect you to have this ridiculously tiny body, and it's a very specific body. But they don't tell you *how* to get it. There is just one idea of the perfect body type, and there were only three things that could happen. Either you were blessed with genetic superiority, like those willowy girls with their long legs who could eat an entire cake and not suffer an additional ounce on the scale; or you could keep weight off through any means possible, including pills, liquid diets, and copious amounts of exercise. The third option wasn't really an option. If you could not achieve the perfect body, then you might as well just quit.

Lucky for me, I had a mentor who was a dear friend of my mother's, and who has proven to be a source of inspiration and strength. She was raised in an abusive household, and as a child she would lock herself in her room and say, "I am not going to be like that." And she couldn't have been more successful. She grew up and created a family that was not only picture-perfect, but just as sweet behind closed doors. She taught me that when we are faced with challenges in life, we can let them define us and hold us down or we can turn them into our greatest strengths. And I was not going to let dance school tell me that I wasn't good enough.

The "Experts" Don't Understand

I would do my best to diet like crazy and eat nothing but steamed chicken and a cracker or two, and my weight would go down, but then it would go right back up. I wasn't very good at starving myself, but I was good at moving my body, so I was usually on a crazy exercise regimen of one kind or another. I got a gym membership, and after eight hours in school I would go and train. My mother scraped together some money that she could barely spare so that I could take Pilates classes. It basically just gave me a massive core, with very overdeveloped abs. Joseph Pilates was a true visionary genius, but his goals are different from mine, and the program did not give me the flat supermodel stomach I was after.

This was a really frustrating cycle for me. I watched my friends damaging their health with rounds of starvation that helped them attain the skinny bodies they were after, and I blamed the school for giving us an unreasonable stereotype to live up to and not providing any real way to achieve it. My weight went up and down, my energy level was a mess, and no matter what I tried, I always slid back to square one. Diets, trainers, the gym—in the end, it was all ineffective. I was a good performer, so my body would dutifully change with each shift in exercise method, but none of them gave me a dancer's body.

Of course, this source of frustration is what would ultimately fuel my search for the solution that the dance professionals, the Pilates professionals, the "experts" at the gym could never give me. Even at school, the counselors had no idea what they were talking about—their obsession with calories actually made me feel *guilty* for eating.

My drive to create a dancer's body from *any kind of body*, not just one that's naturally lean, came from my anger at the system that was basically setting me up to fail. I'm an A+ student who doesn't take F for an answer. If there's an expectation but no solution—well, that's not fair. So a few years later, I would take matters into my own hands.

The end of my dancing career came when I was twenty-two and doing a show in Chicago, complete with regular rounds of major dieting (the chicken and crackers again), and I realized that in order to make it as a dancer, I would never be able to eat again. Since I prefer my plate empty at the end of a meal, not the beginning, I knew a career as a professional dancer was out.

I had no idea what I would do with my life if I wasn't dancing. When my long-distance boyfriend, Eric, came to town and proposed, I said yes.

My First Clue

Eric had back issues that were affecting his basketball career, so during a summer league we found ourselves at a small clinic in Puerto Rico. The doctor's son had a little lizard that he would lead around on a leash. It was definitely not your typical doctor's office.

This doctor had an opinion that was very different from what we had been hearing from all the American doctors. He explained that Eric's injury didn't necessarily mean he needed surgery. In fact, this guy was really against medical intervention. He said, "If you redesign the way that your back muscles are working, and strengthen yourself in a different way, you can cure this."

That was my clue. He was the first person I'd ever heard say that you can do something with your muscles to create change. It made me think about my own struggles with dancing and my weight…This was the first time I asked myself the big question that would change my life: "Can *anyone* have a dancer's body?"

Since I'm a naturally curious person, I started asking questions. Everything the doctor told me, I said, "Why?" and "How?" He showed me all sorts of things, in books, under microscopes. "Look at this," he would say. "Look at how they work. And look at how they change."

Finally I realized that if I did some serious research, I could learn how to really change my own body.

A Decade of Transformation

I dedicated my time to learning and researching everything I could find about muscles. I was on the computer. I was reading books until they were in tatters, and visiting doctors to get the answers that weren't in the books. I was researching exercise and developing my own exercise moves.

While I was pregnant, and later, when I was home with my son Sam, I did so much research on how movement affects the different muscle groups and muscle types that my family thought I was crazy. I was buying books from medical schools, massive stacks of volumes that mapped out the way the muscles fit together and support one another. (My favorite was an anatomy tome published by Taschen called *The Atlas of Human Anatomy and Surgery*.) I talked to neurologists. I talked to sports conditioning doctors. I talked to orthopedic doctors. I made appointments with doctors for sports injuries I didn't really have just so I could have their undivided attention for my curious questions.

Overwhelmingly, the thing I picked up on was how focused all the research was on the large muscle groups, like your biceps, your hamstrings, your quads. All the studies were so focused, in fact, that there was very little information on how to strategically stimulate and utilize the accessory muscles. If it wasn't biceps, if you weren't trying to make it bigger, it was as if it didn't exist. The primary textbooks for physiology training all focused on the large muscle groups. We knew that the accessory muscles existed, but nobody knew why they should care.

It was as if the fitness industry was at a standstill. I felt like the experts were saying: *These are the manuals. There's nothing more to learn.*

That wasn't enough for me, so I kept looking. I already knew that working out the larger muscle groups wasn't the answer. The accessory muscles, I thought, were the key to strengthening and toning the body without bulking up...

Soon after I started implementing what I had learned, I ran into a woman I had known a few years earlier. She couldn't believe how I looked. "Your body's amazing," she kept saying. "I want your arms."

"You know what?" I told her. "You can have them." I started working with her that summer, and by the time September rolled around she didn't have to be jealous of my arms anymore, because hers were more toned and taut than she had ever imagined they could be.

My own transformation took place ten years ago. I gained sixty pounds when I was pregnant with my son, and since I developed this system, I have been exactly the same weight.

Since then, I have helped thousands of women understand how to do the same thing with their bodies. I changed my destiny by learning how to work out properly to get real results, and that's exactly what you'll do with this book. Even if you've been working out for years and nothing seems to help. Even if your body has been resistant to all of today's trendiest regimens, from forms of Pilates to forms of yoga.

My clients are lean and fit. They can manage their weight without excessive dieting. And they're in the best shape they have ever been. Some of them, like Madonna and Gwyneth Paltrow, you've heard of. Some of them, like the woman who had gastric bypass surgery or the career woman with three kids who gained fifty-plus pounds, you haven't. But what they all have in common is this: They have taken control of their lives and their bodies by implementing my workout methods.

Ladies and gentlemen, transformation is possible. And achievable. You can't do it without breaking a sweat, but you can definitely do it.

I am the proof. And in thirty days, with the help of this book, you will be, too.

3

Making Perfect Possible

How the Method Works

When it comes to dresses and heels, trend is everything. But when it comes to exercise, trendier is not better. In fact, in the end, it's useless.

This is what usually happens: Someone jumps on an exercise trend. She sees results in the beginning, because her body is experiencing something new. Give it a month, and she's bummed because she isn't seeing any new results. She talks to friends: "What are you doing?" "Oh my God, I just found the best thing. It's [insert fad here], and I'm seeing results." So she tries the new best thing, and plateaus again, and she has to look for something newer still if she wants more short-term results.

So how do we get long-term results? How do we get to incredible—and stay there?

Trial by Jury

As I already mentioned, my mission has always been to strengthen the smaller muscle groups so that they can pull in the larger muscles, resulting in a lean, long, feminine figure that is not bulky. I knew that I didn't want to *build* upon muscles, I wanted to *pull in* muscles. What my research taught me was that it was all in the accessory muscles. I got really excited, because I knew that these little accessory muscles were like Cinderella muscles. If I could wake them up, I could change anyone. But moving from that realization to a real routine I could share with my clients didn't happen overnight.

In order to develop all of the strategic moves and sequences that make up my Method, I had to go through a lot of trial and error. I used my own body as a test subject, and then I gathered 150 other willing and eager women and put my theories to work.

My ultimate goal was to come up with a small, focused package. You don't try to figure out how to brush your teeth every day: You know how. There's a clear set of directions: Brush for two minutes three times a day, floss, and you're set. You've taken care of your teeth properly, and you don't have to worry that they'll rot and fall out. It's the same with my system: I give you the clear steps. It will take a commitment. But I promise you, you will build a healthy, gorgeous body. You will have beautiful skin tone, tight muscles, and a lot of energy. No more worrying—just results.

The first 150 women I worked with closely were people I knew, and people who had heard about me through word of mouth. My process was very specific. I would carefully measure each woman, and then put her through her paces. Over the five years of trials, I always worked with 150 women. I needed to work with enough women to give me a broad range. I wanted my system to work for everybody, no matter what their age, circumstances, or fitness level. There was the single woman who was stuck at a desk all day and had put on a hundred pounds. The working mom with three kids, ten pounds to lose, and bad skin tone. The twenty-year-old who put all of her paychecks into her body, but still didn't have what she wanted.

Before I started them on the system I had developed through my initial stages of research, I conducted a study to make sure I was right. I didn't want to be 50 percent sure or 75 percent sure. I wanted to be 100 percent positive that what I was teaching was the absolute best way to have a tight, lean, defined body.

So I needed to try *everything*.

Sun and Water

Remember the experiment that you did in the first or second grade? You take two plants and put them in a closet. One gets water and one doesn't. You put two other plants on a windowsill in the sunlight. One gets water and one doesn't. The only plant that survives will be the one that gets everything it needs: water and sunshine. Just water doesn't cut it. Just sunshine doesn't cut it. And of course, as every gardener knows, if you really want a healthy plant, you need to add the right amount of nutrients.

It's the same with my exercise system—the two components work in tandem, supported by the right eating plan—and I proved it through trial and error. First, I had all 150 women try different things. I had some who just did the musculo-structural work, and their cardio would be running. Some just did the musculo-structure, and I let them Spin. And I had some be complete purists to my Method, making sure they did my specific cardio dance aerobics and targeted muscle structure work.

Time and time again, I found that the only program with consistent results was my Method. Doing the muscle work without the right cardio component—substituting running or Spinning, for example—just didn't work effectively. You need the sunshine *and* the water—my special cardio and the muscle reengineering, *as well as* the strategic eating plan to support and speed your progress. If you jump on a trend, the only thing you can be sure of is that you'll be jumping on another one soon. But if you follow my program, integrating the muscle work, the cardio, and the menu—the results you get will be so spectacular, you won't even need to jump on the scale and check.

There were twenty women out of the 150 on the original program who became the basis for my Method. They were the kind who didn't make excuses, who showed up every day, and who really performed. For ninety days, they did the full program, and their results far surpassed those of their peers in the other test groups. These twenty women, with all different backgrounds, shapes, and sizes, all ended up with the same tight, toned, defined body.

Everyone in the other test groups begged to be put on the same program.

That was when I really knew: when everybody wanted in. That was the formula I had been aiming toward. That's when we really got moving.

Refining the Method

Once we had established the basic formula for the Method, it was time to refine it. I worked with 150 women over the course of the next five years, developing and choreographing thirteen new moves every ten days. What I knew, based on my research, was that the accessory muscles wake up fast. They get strong fast. And they get bored fast. So I had to keep them on their toes. In other words, I needed to design a workout that would deliver constant results, so people wouldn't plateau and stop seeing change. By constantly testing new moves, I was able to develop a formula that would work effectively for everybody in the long term. By figuring out the most effective, most strategic moves, I learned how to take any body type and effect a really powerful change.

Every ten days, I would measure the women in the test group and graph the changes in both the large and small muscle groups. As the accessory muscles woke up and started pulling in, the women lost inches and gained confidence. Over time, the empirical evidence from watching them change was so powerful that it drove me to keep working.

After five years, there were sixty people who made it all the way through. Their journey from kindergarten through graduation gave me valuable information about how the weight could stay off and how the definition could remain, despite genetics, old habits, or lifestyle choices.

The results were mind blowing. I was amazed. I was changing women's bodies left and right. It was insanity! In the end, they all had the ideal arms. They all had the ideal butt.

By now, I've done this for so long that my program is foolproof. The Method works for everyone, hands down. So what you'll find in my book is my 30-Day Method: a complete program with a cardio routine, plus new mat exercise sequences every ten days to keep your accessory muscles focused and at attention. You'll lose the fat and tone your muscles. And once you add in the 30-Day eating plan, you'll really see results!

This is a method by which *anyone* can achieve perfection. I promise you, it is possible.

Why My Method Works While the Others Fail

Science is science. Facts are facts. We've always known that the accessory muscles are really powerful when they get stimulated. But until my research, until my moves, nobody had figured out how to keep the accessory muscles stimulated so that the change keeps on happening. With most of the workouts on the market, sooner or later your body will plateau. Since results don't stick, the desire to lose weight remains constant. It's become a chronic problem that never gets solved, except with quick-fix fads. So people come up with the "next new thing." Even the traditional studies have become jumping-off points for trends.

People create these variations because they see how much demand is out there; each fad is a new way to get people into gyms and buying products. But the fact is: Trends don't create long-term results.

When you go from trend to trend to trend, what you feel is your accessory muscles waking up, because you're doing something new. And then they get used to it in a matter of weeks, and they're done working for you. They get bored. They tune out. You stop losing weight.

My Method can beat the plateau. It is a system that is about results, not hope. I use the menus to support your weight loss while you learn how to do the workouts effectively. And I use choreography and muscle work strategically to achieve continuous results, so you look defined instead of massive, and balanced instead of bulky. The gym, the big gym, never gets anyone where they want to be. Do you really want to look like a gym rat? The best thing about people who abuse the gym is that they are, in a way, walking advertisements for my basic message: that we can manipulate our musculostructure to an incredible degree—for worse and better.

Forget Everything They Told You About Exercise

You have more than six hundred muscles in your body. When you go to school to become a personal trainer, or to study exercise physiology, or anything like that, you learn a lot about the major muscles. The biceps work like this. The triceps work like this. A hamstring works like this. Those are our horse muscles, the ones that give us mass and strength. That's all fitness education has traditionally focused on. Nobody in the history of fitness has ever paid attention to the small muscle groups. **And the small muscles are the key.**

During my research, I looked at muscle biopsies to learn how different types of exercise affect muscles. It turns out that different resistance ends up in the muscles in different places: The kind of movement you do affects the kind of muscle that you build. (Remember, you are how you move!)

Even before I took a look through a microscope to see exactly how exercise and resistance change muscle tissue, I knew that working with weights was not the way to go. Weight lifting accomplishes what it sets out to accomplish. It's just not what *I'm* trying to accomplish. When I was a dancer trying to trim down, I worked at a gym with a personal trainer for ages. I was working my butt off and lifting a lot of weights—and I was still forty pounds overweight. My muscles weren't long and lean, they were short and bulky. I looked like I had been tossed into a trash compactor.

If you've ever had a personal trainer, you were probably taught to move your biceps in the linear way they like to move. When you can't feel the action anymore, the weight is upped, and the motion resumes. Same exercise, more weight. When you do this, the weight stresses the muscle to the point that it needs to repair itself, so you're building mass.

I know how much some of you love your little weights, but I'm after a better way.

When you lift weights, you're ripping and repairing the muscle, which builds mass and can ruin your joints and ultimately destroy your skin tone. This is exactly what you don't want. And when you use your own body as resistance, the effects are very similar (and too much Downward Dog can lead to vascular damage, as I've seen with some of my clients).

Weight lifting is not healthy. You're building muscles that are more prone to injury. You're tearing down your joints. You're destroying your structure. And your heart probably isn't happy about it.

Running is terrible for your joints. It makes you work the same muscles over and over again, so you're just strengthening muscles that are already strong enough.

Yoga focuses on legs, abs, and arms—but everything works as its own unit. And some muscles become overdeveloped, while others just waste away, doing nothing.

Tennis might be fun, but it's a prime example of stop-and-go fitness, instead of a balanced cardio workout. It doesn't burn enough energy. It's not a focused enough practice to replace a cardio workout.

My Method tones your muscles and makes you stronger, improving your structure without adding bulk or stressing your joints. It works the entire body as a whole, so you don't end up with big arms and tiny legs, or a massive core and weak arms and legs. And it provides a balance between the muscular restructuring and the cardio, so you end up as fit, sexy, and feminine as you've ever dreamed.

But you have to do it my way.

My Way or the Highway

The human body is like clay, and over the years, through research, trials, and hundreds of success stories, I have learned exactly how to mold it. This is not a trend. This is not a fad. It is a new way of looking at fitness. When you follow my three-part system, you're not just exercising. You're not just burning calories or trying to lose weight. You're doing specific, strategic movements that tone your muscles, improve your skin tone, and combat cellulite. You're becoming fit and energetic, lean and flexible, sexy and feminine.

It *is* possible for you to eat what you want and still have a cellulite-free structure that performs well, is full of energy, and doesn't make you look like you're training for a weight-lifting competition.

Do you want what I have? Do you want what my clients, like Gwyneth, have?

If you're looking for a tight, toned body that is streamlined instead of bulky, it all starts with my 30-Day Method. You won't find it at a gym. You won't find it at a yoga studio or a Pilates mat class. Running, tennis, swimming: nope. If you want to look tight and toned, you need to stop **every other kind of exercise** and **only do my workout.** My promise to you is that if you do what I tell you, you will eventually have the body you've always wanted. Your promise to me is that you will let me redesign your body by 100 percent embracing the system.

This workout is designed to change the way your body is structured. It doesn't matter if you're an athlete, a physicist, or a housewife. Heavy, thin, tall, short: No matter who you are or what your experience level is, I will retrain your body. I do this by working the accessory muscles, the very important ones that nobody pays attention to, in very specific ways. In this program, you'll be pairing this crucial muscle work with cardio and a healthy eating plan. And what you'll see is a transformation.

You're going to hear me using words like *knitting* and *bolting* when I talk about your accessory muscles. These aren't words that are traditionally used when it comes to exercise. But my moves are not traditional. If you want a tight, tiny, trim body, you need to leave behind the repetitive, damaging linear movements, and let me teach your structure to move in angles instead of straight lines. By angles I mean on the diagonal, forward, back, in all directions instead of the more linear up, down, up, of a bicep curl. This is how I wake up your accessory muscles and use them to bolt the larger muscle groups together. By manipulating your structure via strategic muscle exhaustion, tiring out the big muscles so the accessory muscles can activate and strengthen, I can knit your muscles together to give you definition and strength.

When I talk about knitting, I mean that you'll be pulling and tightening your muscles together to make them more compact, as opposed to bigger. *Knitting* isn't a scientific term—it's an analogy for the unique way we're going to tighten and tone. By bolting, I mean gathering a collection of muscles around a joint—or contracting them—in several specific areas, as if you're literally fusing your muscles together to improve and renew your shape. The moves work to bolt the muscles in these key places to lift the glutes, firm the outer thighs, contract around the hip flexors, and connect all the muscles in your upper body so they pull up and in—and believe me, you are going to notice the difference!

The Designer Body

I consider myself a designer. If you embrace my program, you're inviting me to re-create your body. It's like organic plastic surgery—I am literally reshaping the figure that you have into the one that you want. If you were visiting a plastic surgeon—someone who uses a knife to reshape—you would trust his or her vision. You wouldn't go to two plastic surgeons at once—you'd end up looking like a Picasso, with your nose on your forehead. Maintaining your other exercise while you do my program interferes with my design.

Since you are how you move, as we've discussed, I can't have any other surgeons in the operating room with me, so to speak. If you're reading this book, you've already invited me in. Now you need to trust me.

That is why I ask you to totally focus on all three components of my system during these first thirty days.

Commitment = Results

This is not the same old fitness book with a different cover. My system is designed so that you will never become static. Static is what causes plateaus. Static is why you sweat in a gym and still don't get the results you want. Static is why you're constantly searching for a new solution to the same old problem.

But you need to be honest if you want it to work. I can try to motivate you, and I can give you the tools—but you're the one who will have to be ready to get rid of all of the excuses. I've seen it time and time again with my clients. Someone will come in just swearing that she's doing my program perfectly, but isn't seeing the results she wants. Of course, since I know the Method works, I'm always digging to discover why it's not working for someone.

"Oh, I swear to you I'm doing the menus," she'll say. But when I push, it's suddenly, "Oh, but I had a handful of this." Or, "I always do the whole workout!" And when I say, "Really?" I'll hear, "Well, I came to my workout, but my daughter called me seven times during it, so I didn't really finish."

You know how it goes, right? Well, it needs to stop right now. If you want to see results, you need to commit 100 percent for the next thirty days. Think about it this way: Isn't it worth a month of your time to change the rest of your life?

That's why I'm asking you to show up every day. Think of the next thirty days as a boot camp. Be present, be real. I will ask you to exercise at least an hour a day. To follow the menus. To be true to yourself and your goals. You can attain perfection if you use the tools that I am giving you. You can have a body more beautiful than you ever dreamed.

But you can't just do it once and think you're going to look that great. You have to build a new habit, a new framework. You need to do this every day: every, single day. The results will be worth the thirty-day sacrifice, I guarantee it!

And there's no better time to start than today. So let's get started.

PART TWO

GETTING KICK-STARTED

4

Making the Method Work for You

How to Give—and Get—100 Percent

By now you know you're about to completely change the way your body looks and feels. In order to do this, you have to stop thinking of fitness as a hobby, and make it a priority. Every element of the program is integral, and you should regard each one as pivotal to your success.

It is the *correct combination* of the three Method elements—muscle work, cardio, and menus—that is going to drive your complete transformation. If you overdo the dieting but don't rebuild your structure, you're going to be what I call "skinny fat." If you overdo the structure work but don't do the cardio, you're going to have a layer of fat hiding your new physique. And if you overdo the cardio—and don't balance it out with the structure redesign—you're going to have loose, hanging skin that will *not* look good in a bikini.

The goal of this boot camp is to shock your muscles, reinvigorate your system, and redesign your body. The Muscle Design and the Cardio Complement, along with the 30-Day Kick-Start Menus, work together to help you create the body you've always dreamed of having. But it's like any good recipe: If you skip a step, there's no way it's going to come out tasting like the chef intended.

If you're dedicated to the muscle work but skimp on your cardio, you're going to have the tight muscles, but you're also going to feel blubbery on the surface because the fat has nowhere to go. If you do too much cardio, or crash-diet, and don't do the muscular structure work, then your skin is going sag, because you've had a rapid weight loss but no muscle transformation. You're going to look like a sharpei when you're naked. But if you do everything in the right balance, then the muscular structure changes. The fat is burned. And the skin will come back to the muscle. The skin is the last thing to make a change, but it will.

If you get yourself past the beginner's level, and you really learn to perform, this boot camp will help you look and feel fantastic.

It's All About You

Now that you understand what the 30-Day Method is and how it works, let's talk about how to make it work best for *you*. If you approach your training like an amateur, you will not get the results you want. If you approach it like a professional, your muscles will become taut and toned; your structure will be redefined and redesigned.

What does it take to be a professional? It requires commitment. It means getting rid of all the excuses. You'll need to pick a set time to exercise and dedicate a space to your program, even if that means that you have to move your couch three feet to the left every day. And along the way you'll get to know yourself, embrace your true potential, and learn to be your best critic. All these things are part of what it takes to move forward, to restructure your structure, to achieve a level of perfection you have only dreamed about.

You will show up every day. You will try your hardest. And you will do it right.

Real achievement will come through four steps:

1. Schedule your program.
2. Prepare the environment.
3. Connect to yourself.
4. Push yourself.

Step One: Schedule Your Program

My 30-Day Method isn't going to be your new hobby: It's going to be your new job. In order to fully commit to this boot camp, you have to commit to it in your mind—and you have to put it in your calendar. You'll need to set aside forty-five minutes to one and a half hours each day, depending on your fitness level, your strength, and your commitment.

When I am training someone over a long period, I do not recommend exercising every day—we all deserve a day off. But the kick-start program is different. This is a thirty-day program of transformation that requires you to show up and sweat *every day*.

Think back to the last time you began a job at a new company. As soon as you accepted the position, your new managers established your schedule and responsibilities, letting you know exactly when you needed to be there and what you needed to be doing. Wherever your new job took you—to an office, a retail shop, a school—when you were on the premises, you were there to do one thing…work. The same goes for this program. When the scheduled time for your workout arrives, that is the only thing that you should do. The allotted hours are not the time to read a magazine, do the dishes, or help your son with his homework. This is not the time to make to-do lists, eat an apple, or answer the phone. Everything must be left outside the room: your family responsibilities, your professional responsibilities, and any last-minute household chores short of real, actual emergencies. (Fighting a fire is an emergency. Finding your daughter's favorite jeans for her is not.)

Consistency Is Key

Many people ask me what the best time is for exercise. The answer is: the time that works best for you. I encourage my clients to *pick their time* and *stick to it*. You need to block out a *consistent* time in your schedule, whether it's in the morning, the afternoon, or the evening.

There are a few things to take into consideration when you set up your schedule. First of all, what time of day do you perform the best? Morning people who jump out of bed ready to take on the world should work out in the early-morning hours. Night people who sleep until noon and then become energized and upbeat after 9 p.m. should exercise in the evening.

You'll need to consider your other responsibilities along with natural temperament. We all have busy lives. What time of the day are you least likely to have interruptions? If you're a morning person, but you're also a parent getting kids off to school by 7 a.m., there's no way you'll be able to focus during the regular morning bustle. If you're a night person, but you're also a professional who works extremely long hours, the odds that you'll want to put on your sneakers when you stagger in the door at 10:30 p.m. are slim.

Excuses get in the way of your success, so when you lay out your schedule, be firm and be realistic. Block out the time.

Step Two: Prepare the Environment

You've invested in this book, in reading it, in your time, in your commitment. Get to the next level by preparing the right environment for working out correctly. No matter what your home looks like, you can make it happen. If, like most people, you don't have room to create a home gym, create a temporary space that you can dismantle after you're done with your workout for the day. If you have to change a playroom into your boot camp room, do it. If you have to change an office, do it. If you have to move furniture each day, do it.

1. Select a room with hardwood floors, if you have it, for the Cardio Complement. (If you don't, it's okay.)

2. Gather your equipment. You'll need **sneakers,** a **mirror,** and a **yoga mat** for the first ten-day sequence. For the second ten-day sequence, you're going to incorporate a sturdy **chair.** When your strength increases, you'll add **light ankle weights.**

3. Keep the room warm. You can't have the air-conditioning blasting. It should be a warm room, in the eighties, because I want you to sweat.

Step Three: Connect to Yourself

In order to correctly perform the series I will be teaching you, you need to be uninhibited in your movements and committed to doing this right. I need you to really connect yourself to this process. Dance aerobics alone won't do it. Raising

What You Need

You do not need any fancy equipment to achieve amazing results with this 30-Day Method Kick Start.

Sneakers: A good pair of sneakers is imperative for avoiding injury. Get a new pair if your current kicks are in less-than-stellar condition. For dance aerobics, you'll want shoes that are light, breathable, and have proper support. (No Keds, skate sneakers; or fashion-plate sneakers. Athletic shoes only!) Personally, I love Nike Shox and Mizuno Inspires. A pair of socks is also key.

Mirrors: Get three cheap mirrors at your local hardware store and line them up in front of you.

Mat: If you don't have a yoga mat, use a towel.

Chair: Use a regular kitchen or dining chair. Choose an armless chair, since you'll use the seat for doing your moves, and one with a back that you can use as a barre for balance. Make sure it's sturdy and secure—you'll be putting your full weight on it, and you don't want to worry about it toppling over.

and lowering your arms on cue won't do it. You can't just *do* it. You have to *perform* it.

You can raise your arms in the air and not be doing anything. And you can raise your arms in the air and actually be engaging in your workout. If you aren't properly connected, your results aren't going to be what they could be. If you really connect, the results are going to blow you away.

As you know, you are engaging the accessory muscles, those behind-the-scenes muscles, and in order to do so correctly you must have the power to exhaust the muscles that want to do the movements in the first place. You have to exhaust the star performers. Your larger muscles, the ones you hear about all the time— biceps, triceps, hamstrings, et cetera—they want to do the work. They're used to doing the work. You need to engage the smaller muscles, the ones that usually

Be Self-Centered!

I once had a woman walk out of one of my classes. This had never happened before, and I'm very sensitive to feedback from my students, spoken or unspoken, so I asked some of the people in the class, "Does anybody know why she left?" One girl said, "Yeah. She turned to me and said, 'All she does is stare at herself in the mirror the whole time. I'm leaving.'" She thought that I was being vain, but I was just watching myself carefully. I wasn't looking at my hair, or my workout gear. I was watching my moves, making sure my performance was accurate.

That's what I need you to do. I need you to be completely absorbed in yourself. One hundred percent focused on yourself and your performance.

---

get a free ride. In order to wake up the accessory muscles, though, you have to have a presence. You have to perform. You have to be connected, and you have to care about the movements.

The best way to do that is to really focus on yourself. That's why we work with the mirrors. I am a huge fan of mirrors. Part of connecting with yourself is seeing yourself as you really are. There's a big difference between thinking you're doing something, and actually doing something. In order to be successful with your at-home exercise program, you need to be your own critic.

Are you watching yourself when you do the moves? Are you doing them correctly, feeling them, pursuing them, really showing up? Or are you just going through the motions? Focus on *connection*.

In the following pages, I'm going to teach you a connection exercise that should be performed before you do your daily stretching routine and launch into the sequence of the day.

When I teach my classes, I'm like a director. If my students aren't doing my leg lift in the right way, it bothers me, because the movements are part of a performance. Imagine a corps of dancers. The one who does it wrong ruins the show. And it isn't just about going left when everyone else goes left. It's about performing the moves with intention as much as accuracy.

By really connecting with yourself and your intention, you will give yourself room to perform, which will make every move count.

Step Four: Push Yourself

I'm not Tinker Bell. I say this all the time in my classes. People want me to be Tinker Bell. They want the fairy dust. But there is no fairy dust. Only you, your commitment, and the workout. Somehow, we've begun to equate the American dream with always feeling comfortable. We've gotten soft. We want the feel-good-now, fix-me-now, perfect abs in five minutes a day. But it doesn't work like that.

In the beginning, you'll feel uncomfortable. You'll feel sore. But as you go through the sequences, day by day, your muscles are going to react, and your accessory muscles are going to wake up, and the power that you develop is going to amaze you.

You can't just count on me to change you. I'm going to give you the tools, but you are the one who has to do the work. You're going to change, but you have to do your part.

Sweat is the only fairy dust.

That's why I need you to sweat every day during the 30-Day Method. Every single day. Sweat is key. It has value because of what it does for your muscles, and because it has intense detoxifying benefits. Sweat leads to weight loss. So many people say, "Oh, it's just water weight." Well, water weight, when you get to your goal, can make or break how you feel.

You want to sweat every day. You want to get your body to a point where you can achieve maximum results, and the only way to do that is to work it.

Throughout the program, your body is being challenged by repetition, challenged by angle, challenged by rotation. It's challenged by its own weight, by choreography, by connection. And once you get good at it, it's challenged by opposing forces.

Exercise: Discovering the Cross-Vectors of Force

Your body is full of energy and power. Everyone's body has so much energy, but most people have no idea how to access it. As soon as you wake up that power, and learn how to use it and direct it and push it and pull it, you are going to completely transform the way you look and feel.

Part of pushing yourself is making sure that you're using all your power when you execute each move. What we're after is harnessing what I call the cross-vectors of force. For example:

> Lift up your right hand and reach it out as if you've dropped your most prized possession. Your great-grandmother's diamond engagement ring has fallen through a hole in the wall. It's over there, somewhere. And your arm can fit through the hole, but just up to your shoulder. So you're really extending that arm out, reaching as far and as hard as you can, but the wall is holding your shoulder back.
>
> Now let's say you want to reach farther, but you're afraid you're going to fall through the wall. So you ask your best friend to hold your arm on the other side. That action, stretching both ways at once, activates the cross-vector force.

If you focus on that picture, you're going to feel the power running through you. Every time I do a leg movement, my hip is going in the opposite direction. When I stretch my right arm to the right, I'm pulling to the left with the other side. It always works with the motion. You're going to extend out, reach beyond, and then pull it all back in. And then you reach it all out, and then you pull it all back in.

The repetition of pulling and relaxing sends little vibrations through your muscles, and the vibrations are what will tighten and tone. Instead of creating strength through mass, you create strength through unity. As we discussed, if you work a muscle over and over with a deadweight, you're just ripping muscle fibers and repairing, and ripping and repairing. Here it's a totally different action. With the cross-vectors of force, instead of rip and repair, which builds mass on top of muscle, we are tightening the muscle from the inside. We're getting rid of

Don't Fall into the Reward Trap

When you're doing an at-home program, you have to learn to be your own teacher, and your own critic, and hold yourself accountable. I want you to be proud of yourself for the effort you're putting into changing your body. But I don't want you to become too proud too soon. Five leg reps isn't going to do it. Ten minutes of cardio isn't going to do it. When you start justifying why five reps of each exercise is really great, when you start to reward yourself too soon, you start to sabotage your progress. This won't get results and won't get you to the next level.

You need to push yourself to the next level. There's a difference between believing in yourself and rewarding yourself. I am constantly encountering people who think that an ice cream cone is a great reward for a good workout. Well, unless you've hit your goal, it's not the time yet. That's what boot camp is. You work hard until you reach your goal. You do not reward yourself just for lacing up your sneakers.

Later on, you'll be able to be less regimented about what you eat and still maintain your beautiful physique with exercise. But in the 30-Day boot camp stage, it is very important that you focus on your goals and continuously push yourself. You can do it!

the space and pushing the fat to the surface, where the cardio will melt it away.

With my program, you'll use the cross-vectors of force to shrink and tighten your muscles. You'll then use the Cardio Complement to help burn off all that fat. Ultimately, your skin—which is the very last thing to regain elasticity, but it will— will bind tightly to your muscle, to give you the toned look you want. If you stick with the program and recalibrate your body to function effectively and get rid of the excess fat, you'll maintain your new shape and have the body you've always dreamed of.

In other words, you'll become a high-performance machine.

5

Connecting Your Body and Mind

Daily Connection Exercises and Stretches

First things first, remember—each time you exercise, turn

off your phone or computer so you aren't distracted by the outside world. This is your time to do something for *yourself,* not your time to do things for others. When you're ready, you're going to preface the Muscle Design Work and the Cardio Complement with a connection exercise and a stretching sequence. After your focus is aligned and your muscles are warmed up, then you'll begin.

Connect

Once you have disconnected from the world at large, it is time to mentally engage yourself—to connect to your body and shut everything else out. Focus. You've already made this commitment to the time that you have set aside for yourself, for your body—so make sure that it's actually not a waste of your time.

So many people waste their time exercising. They don't concentrate. They watch TV or read. Their phone is still ringing and they are still distracted—which makes exercise time a stop-and-go sport. And stop-and-go sports, or stop-and-go activities, will not change your body. So if you're serious about changing your body, and you're serious about getting the most out of your workout, then take this time to focus.

The following visualization exercise will connect your brain to your body. By being connected and striving for total control over your muscles, you will learn to access the cross-vectors of force, which are so powerful, but so difficult to get in tune with.

This 30-Day Kick Start is not just about seeing amazing results quickly. It's also about laying the groundwork and the foundation for success for the rest of your life.

Your Daily Connection Exercise

Look at yourself in the mirror, and say your name. Say your name like you're happy. Say your name like you're sad. Say your name like you just met the president. Say your name like you've just been pooped on by a bird. Say your name ten times, without moving. No flipping your hair, making a funny face, rolling your eyes. Just be completely relaxed and present, look yourself in the eye, and repeat your own name.

Learning how to relax while doing something unfamiliar is going to help you improve your performance, which is going to get you the results you want, faster. Taking this time to connect to your body—just mentally connect, just taking a few moments to shut everything else out so that you are able to focus—is going to completely change the effectiveness of your session performance.

Your Daily Stretching Sequence

It is really important that before you start the Muscle Design or the Cardio Complement, you take the proper time to do the following five warm-up moves.

Stretching before a workout helps get the energy moving through your muscles, and it warms the muscles. When you get your muscles warm, they respond more to the movements. It's like warming clay before you mold it. (That's why I don't like a cold room.)

The Right Amount of Stretch

You don't want to spend hours stretching. Overstretching can be dangerous. You want the muscles to be flexible, but you also want them to be quick to perform, and you want them to be powerful. Muscles that are too flexible (overstretched) are not. If you focus only on flexibility, and not on strength and power, you tend not to have the skin tone benefits that come from working the muscles and strengthening the muscles. There needs to be a balance. I don't want you to push your flexibility to the point where you don't have a muscle that contracts as easily as it flexes. Still, I do want you to warm up your muscles.

These simple stretching exercises will open your hips in the proper places. They will stretch out your hip flexors, so the muscles will bolt to the lower abs and flatten. These warm-up stretches will open up your hips in a way that should feel freeing to you. If you still feel like your hip flexors are tight, you can do these stretching exercises at the end of your workout, too.

Once you become proficient in the muscle work and cardio, you will be ready to add ankle weights. The stretching at that point becomes even more important. It's very dangerous to add a weight at the end of your leg without warming it up beforehand. That's when injury happens. So no matter how good you get at the work, don't cut out the stretching. And of course, before you begin this or any other exercise or diet program, you should consult your health care professional.

TA Method Daily Stretches

Stretch #1: Flowing Triangle Stretch

Stance: Stand with your feet about three feet apart, and then rotate your right foot out so your heel is directly in line with the arch of your left foot.

Action: Reach your right hand down toward the floor. If you can't reach the floor, rest your right hand on the top of your foot, your ankle, or your shin. The stretch comes from reaching your left arm all the way up toward the ceiling so your arms form a straight line.

The cross-vectors of force applied: When you do the Flowing Triangle, you'll immediately engage the cross-vectors of force for maximum efficiency. As you press your right hand into the ground and reach your left arm up, you want to feel as if you are being pulled apart. Your right hand is being pressed down through the floor, your left arm is being pulled up through the ceiling.

Flow: Come down into the stretch, and come right back up. As you rise up, you're going to place your hands on your hips and let the momentum draw your ribs past your left hip. You should feel a hamstring stretch as well as a slight stretch in your groin.

Reps: Four times on the right, and then switch sides. Rotate the left foot out, left hand on the ground, right hand in the air, and repeat four times.

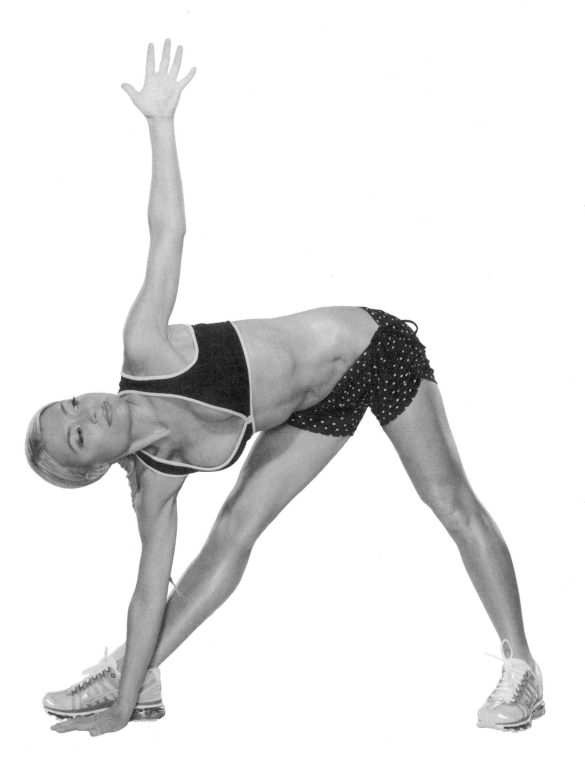

Stretch #2: Plié Stretch

Stance: Rotate both of your feet out to the sides, wider than shoulder width apart.

Action: Bend into a deep plié or squat position, placing your elbows on your knees.

Flow: Rock back and forth from side to side, feeling the stretch in your inner thighs.

Reps: Repeat for up to one minute.

Stretch #3: Thigh and Hip Stretch

Stance: Begin in plié position.

Action: Shift all of your weight over your left foot so your right leg is straight and your left leg is in a deep bend, then flex your right foot, toes pointing to the ceiling.

Flow: Shift to the other side, so your right leg bends and your left leg is straight with toes flexed and pointing to the ceiling. Rotate your feet forward, and drop your head to the ground. Straighten your legs and roll up.

Reps: Repeat for about a minute.

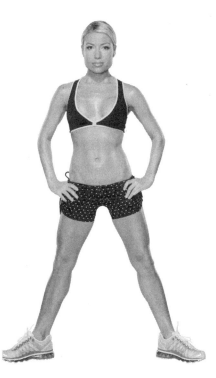

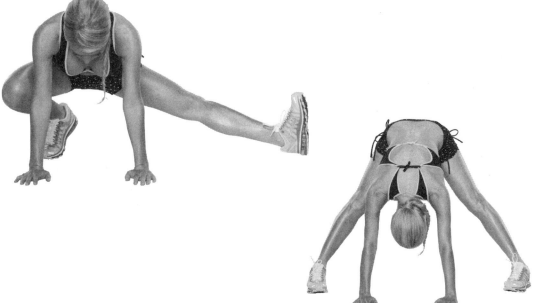

Stretch #4: Side Stretch

Stance: Stand with your feet together.

Action: Reach your right arm over your head and bend to the left. Wrap your left arm around your back and hold on to your right hip.

Flow: Start when you bend your right arm, and reach deeper into the stretch until you are reaching so far to the side that your right arm straightens. Then switch to the other side.

Reps: Repeat for about a minute.

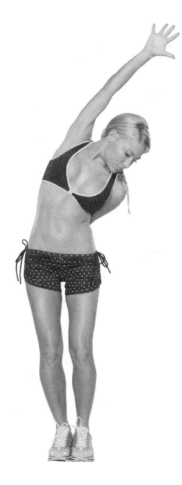

Stretch #5: Hands to Floor Stretch

Stance: Stand with your feet together.

Action: Roll down and touch the floor.

Flow: Bend your knees, then stretch up, repeating the flow and then rolling up when you are finished with the stretch.

Reps: Repeat for about a minute.

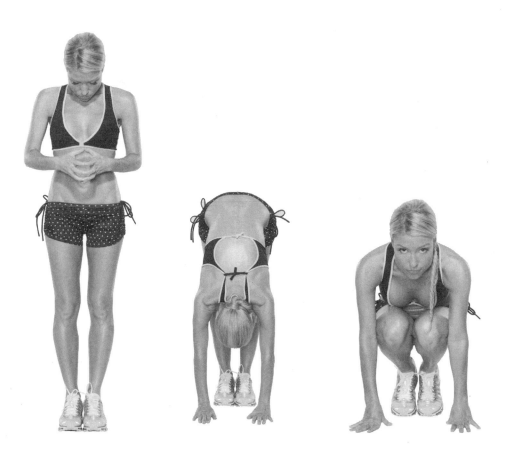

PART THREE

TRACY ANDERSON'S
30-DAY METHOD

6

TA Method Muscle Design

Your Three 10-Day Muscle Work Sequences

By now you know that TA Muscle Design comprises three

sequences that will last for ten days each. Each sequence is made up of sixteen targeted moves that work your arms, your abs, and your legs. In order to keep the accessory muscles activated and stop them from getting bored (causing you to plateau), it is necessary to begin the next sequence of moves every ten days.

You will notice that on days 1, 11, and 21, your muscles will become exhausted quickly. Each day that follows those initial days, you will notice your muscles developing an ease with the movements. Day 5 will be easier than day 3. Day 15 will be easier than day 12. Each time you change over to the next sequence, you will be learning new moves that will challenge your body in a new way, and your body will have to work to master the new movements. By doing this, you keep your accessory muscles awake so that your transformation can be continuous.

Reps

On the very first day that you begin the Method Muscle Design, I want you to do only twenty reps of every exercise. If you cannot do twenty reps, that's fine. You're going to work up to it, and beyond. I want you to push yourself, but I don't want you to hurt yourself. It's a fine balance.

If you feel the burn at ten reps, don't be too quick to pat yourself on the back and move on. Keep going. See how far you can really get.

If you can do twenty reps the first day, I want you to keep setting goals for your-self. The next day is going to be twenty-five. The day after that, thirty. Ultimately, I want you to get to a maximum of sixty reps.

If you can do sixty reps for three days in a row, then you can add the ankle weights. Only add ankle weights when you can, with perfect form, hit all the reps with no break.

With ankle weights, never go above forty reps, because I don't want you to become overexhausted. Again, it's a balance.

Doing It Right (and Left)

In the photos and on the DVD, I'm generally doing the moves on my right side. Make sure you repeat the same move on the left side! When you're working your arms, I want you to do *all* the moves in the sequences for arms on the right side, and then all the moves on the left side. This helps to tire out the big muscles so that you can really activate your accessory muscles and see faster results.

Sequence 1: Days 1–10

Welcome to Sequence 1, a ten-day program that is designed to be both manageable and challenging. The first ten days are all about your body learning to work in a way that isn't instinctual. You're forcing the big guys—the big muscles—to take a backseat so the backstage muscles—the accessory muscles—can step into the spotlight. The reps and the sequencing are designed to get to the large muscle groups, exhaust them, and then have the small muscle groups wake up and become engaged.

Be prepared: The first and second days of Sequence 1, you can expect to feel almost like you have the flu. It won't be the usual kind of area-specific soreness, like "My abs are really feeling it," or "My arms are really sore." It's an all-over-tired feeling. When you cause friction within the muscular fibers, as you'll be doing with my Method, it's different from repairing muscular fibers. It feels different. You'll experience an everywhere soreness.

Once you get past the first two days, you'll start to crave the pain. I know that sounds crazy, but it's true. By day 3, your body will begin to respond very quickly—and it will want more. This is where the addiction kicks in, and then you'll start to see results very quickly.

By day 10, you'll be able to do everything that I'm asking you. And then your body is ready for the next step.

But before we get ahead of ourselves, let's begin with the first step. Or rather, the first kick back. Remember, the goal is to work up to a maximum of sixty reps.

Getting Started

You're going to do moves 1–7 all on your right side and then switch to your left. After you finish the four crunch moves, begin your arm exercises the same way you did your leg and butt exercises—all on your right side first, so you really get at those accessory muscles, and then all on the left side. This pattern will repeat throughout the sequences. Right side first for legs and butt, then left side for legs and butt. Right side first for arms, then left side for arms.

Move #1: Bend and Kick Back

This exercise will challenge your balance and encourage you to engage your cross-vectors for increased stability.

Stance: Kneel on your hands and knees. Place both hands firmly on the floor in front of you, shoulders squared to the front of the room.

Action: Shift your weight to your arms and extend your right leg directly behind your right hip on an upward diagonal, toes pointed, so that your body extends in a long line from your chest back through your leg. Then your knee travels forward toward your right shoulder. Keep your leg at hip height even as it bends at ninety degrees.

Flow: Extend your leg back and above behind you, then bring your knee forward toward your shoulder. After your reps, repeat on the other side.

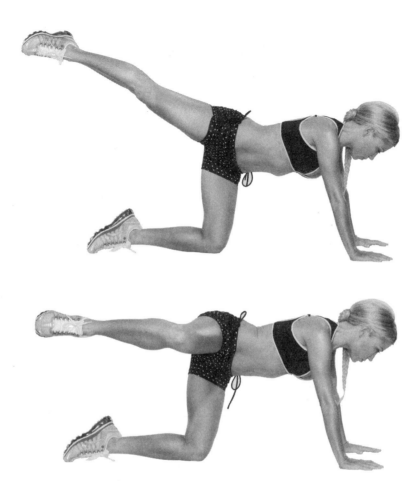

Engaging the cross-vectors: The flow of this move relies on stretch as well as the cross-vector forces. The stretch helps to make your muscles more pliable…as you lean forward, you are stretching your large muscle groups. As you lift your leg and it travels back—that's when the cross-vectors kick in. When I do this move, the energy moves forward through my right hip, which reaches forward, along with my upper body and chest. Then everything recoils. The leg moves back, the upper body and chest move forward, and the cross-vector begins to affect your accessory muscles.

Move #2: Side Hip Straight Leg Lift

The Side Hip Straight Leg Lift begins to cinch the muscles in a strategic way to give you that perfect butt.

Stance: Begin by kneeling on all fours. Place your right foot out to the side, leg straight, in line with your hip. Foot and knee point forward.

Action: Lift your right leg up to the side until it reaches about two inches above the hip. As you raise the leg up, you are also moving it to the right, while the left glute (butt muscle) pulls in the opposite direction. The cross-vector of force travels through both glute muscles, bolting through both of them.

Flow: Lift up and down. Up and down. The challenge here is not to plop your leg down on the ground. So when you raise it up, you also want to guide it down, just touch your big toe on the ground, and then lift it up again. Then you'll really feel the engagement in the glute of your nonworking leg.

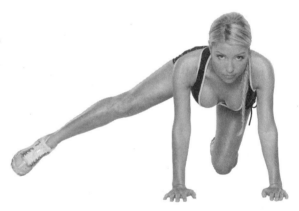

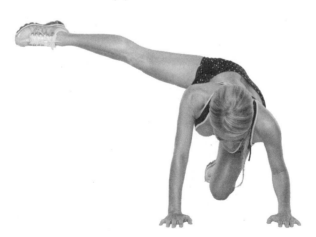

Move #3: Frog Cross Leg Lift

You can work the cross-vectors here in two ways—just don't forget to have fun!

Stance: Lie down on your left side, supporting yourself with your left arm. Place your right hand on your right hip.

Action: Cross your right foot in front of your left foot, stretching your body long, and then bring your crossed ankles in toward your butt, bending your legs so the right knee is pointing toward the ceiling and the left knee is pointing toward the front of the room. Once your feet are as close to your butt as you can get them, extend your right leg to the ceiling and your left leg out to the right side. Then bend the legs back into the "frog" position (ankles crossed), and finish by extending your legs back out to the side.

Flow: As you move through this sequence, reach your right arm forward for balance as the leg extends toward the ceiling, then bring it back to your hip. The goal is to always keep your hips stacked. Make sure to execute the movements in a smooth, controlled manner. Extend all the way through your legs when they straighten, and try to turn your right leg out to its maximum rotation while keeping your hipbones pointing forward.

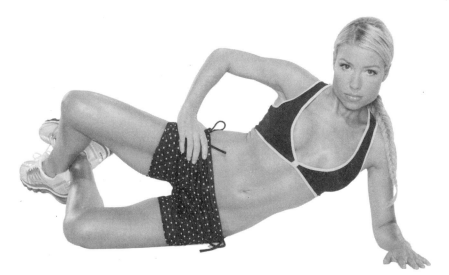

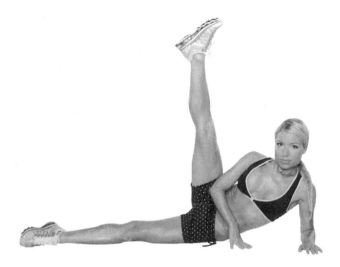

Maximizing Cross-Vectors

The cross-vectors of force here happen in two places. When you are working the right side, I want your right hand on your hip to remind you to keep your hip forward while your right knee moves back. (You can return your hand to the ground for balance if you need to.) That's one cross-vector, which you'll feel twisting across your quadriceps—exactly how those large muscle groups don't want to work. Conventional forms of fitness would ask you to move your leg forward and back, in the way that feels most natural. But when you move with the cross-vectors, you feel it pulling across your quads (along the front of the thigh).

The cross-vector on the kick up is also really important. Your bottom leg must be awake and active. When you are working your right leg, you should feel the left leg reaching away from your left shoulder.

When lying on the mat, you'll feel the energy of pulling in two directions all the way down your torso. You are not just lounging around watching television, moving one leg. Feel the energy. You're here, aren't you? So let's do it right.

Move #4: Diagonal Knee Touchdown and Leg Extension

This move takes a diagonal approach to reach your accessory muscles. One of the most effective elements of this exercise is the cross-vector activity that occurs when the leg travels.

Stance: Lie on your left side, supporting yourself with your left arm. Bend both legs to attitude position by pulling your knees forward so your feet stay in line with your hips and torso.

Positive Attitude

You'll often hear me say to hold your legs in **attitude** position. *Attitude* is a dance term that means your leg is turned out with the knee bent at about a ninety-degree angle.

Action: Raise your right leg, maintaining the bend in the knee on both legs, and reach forward with your right knee to tap the ground in front of you, just around mid-thigh. Bring the heel of your top leg as close as you can toward your butt as you bring the knee forward to tap the ground. Then stretch the leg back behind you and up, at a diagonal.

Kick Like You Mean It

If you just kick your leg up, you aren't going to be accomplishing anything. If you make sure that the hip comes forward and the heel comes up and back on the kick—feeling your glute (butt muscle) engage—you're going to be activating my design, and transforming your body.

Flow: Tap your knee, bring your leg back behind you and up, on a diagonal, and then repeat. Down, tap, back, and up. Down, tap, back, and up.

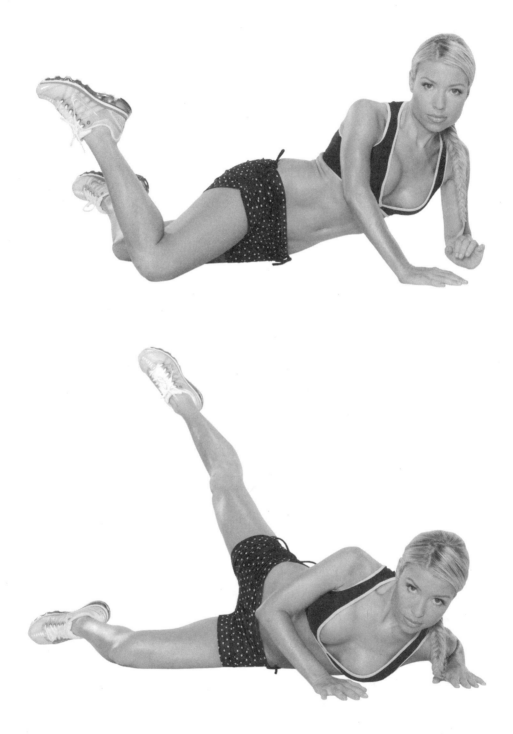

Move #5: Three Beats, One Lift

The cross-vector here is easy to access. When you lift, make sure that you're stretching your top leg up toward the ceiling while your bottom leg reaches to the floor.

Stance: Lie on your left side with your left forearm on the ground. Right hand is on your hip or on the floor in front of you for stability. Stretch your legs long on the mat. Feet are pointed.

Action: We're going to use a three-part, one-beat lift for this move. Begin by moving your right foot in front of your left foot, then arcing it over your left leg and behind, then arcing it back to the front. For the lift, flex your foot and lift your leg straight up into the air...the right leg is turned out for this move.

Flow: Front, back, front, lift. Front, back, front, lift.

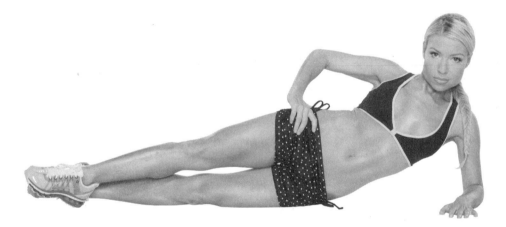

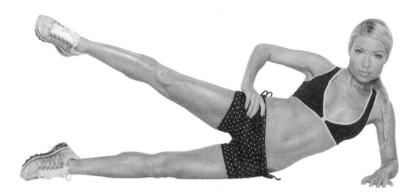

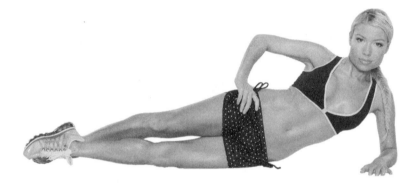

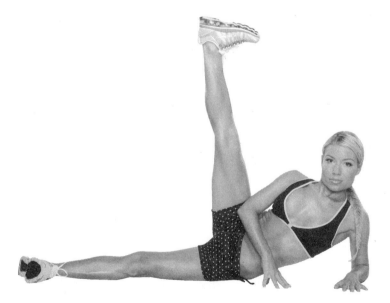

Move #6: Diagonal Up and Back

The cross-vector here is another really important one, but it's a twisting one. As your right leg goes up and behind you, the left hip pulls down in a front diagonal to the right, in the opposite direction.

Stance: Begin by kneeling. Place your right foot out to the side, leg straight, in line with your hip. Foot points forward. Place your hands on the floor under your shoulders in front of you so that you're on all fours with your leg stretched out to the side.

Action: Lift your leg to the side and bend it ninety degrees. Then you're going to move it so that it travels back behind you, beyond the left shoulder, beyond the left hip. Then straighten it out behind you. Bring the leg back to the right side (bending through) and release the leg down to the floor, contracting through your lower abs.

Flow: Up, reach to straighten, and down. Up, reach to straighten, and down.

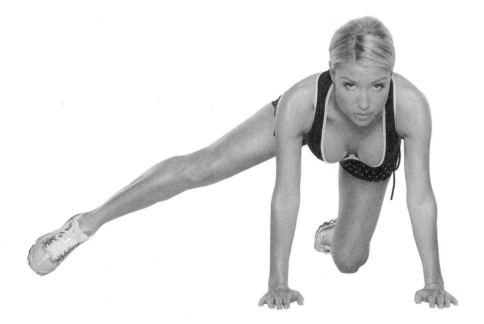

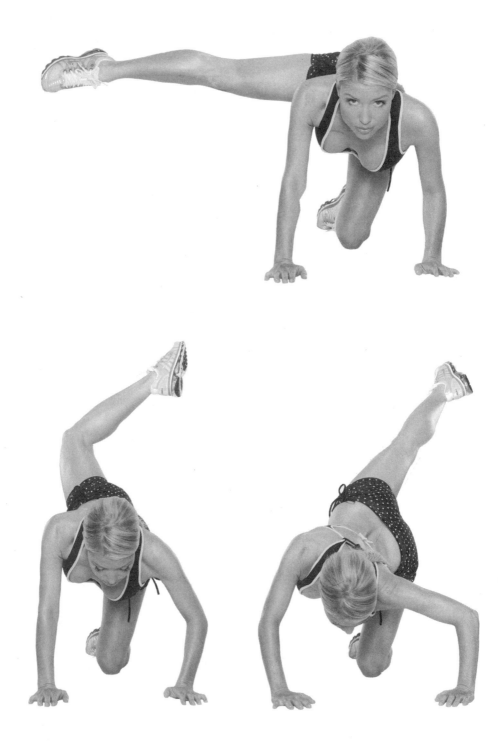

Move #7: Attitude Butt Lift

When I say attitude, I don't just mean "with bent knee." Every move must be executed with style and precision. Remember, this is a performance.

Stance: Start on your hands and knees. Cross your right shin over your left calf.

Action: Lift the right leg back in an attitude, kicking your leg straight at the top, then return through an attitude to crossed legs.

Flow: Lift, kick, and return.

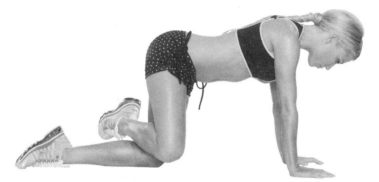

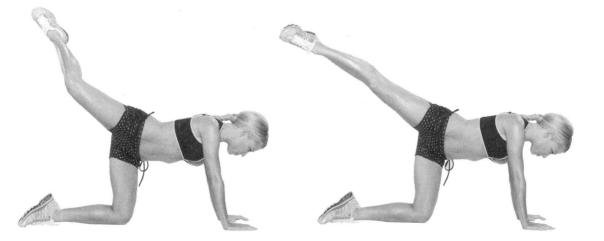

Move #8: Straight Leg Crunches

Women should never do crunches with their knees up. It's much more effective for a flat stomach, and not an overdeveloped rectus abdominus, to do it with legs straight out.

Stance: Lie on your mat with your legs straight out in front of you, and your hands behind your head. Legs are together, and toes are pointed.

Action: Lift your head and your shoulders, contracting your abdominals, and then relax onto the floor. Legs remain on the floor.

Flow: Crunch up and down, up and down.

Crunching Numbers

Eventually, you'll be able to do eighty of these. When you're getting started, it's okay to just do ten and take a rest—although making it to twenty is even better.

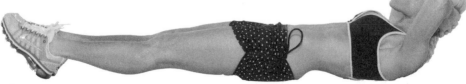

Move #9: Crunches with Attitude Lifts

Alternating legs helps activate the muscles for a sleeker torso.

Stance: Lie on your mat with your legs straight out in front of you, hands behind your head. Legs are together, and toes are pointed.

Action: Crunch up like you just did in the Straight Leg Crunches while simultaneously lifting your right leg to the ceiling in a turned-out attitude position (knee bent at a ninety-degree angle), then place it back on the floor. Switch to the left leg.

Flow: Crunch and right leg up, and down. Crunch and left leg up, and down.

Activating the cross-vectors in Crunches with Attitude Lifts takes a bit of focus. When you crunch up and your head moves forward, your knee twists out to the side, sparking a small cross-vector around each hip flexor (a muscle in your hip joint). And of course, when you lie back down, your toes should be moving in the opposite direction of your head.

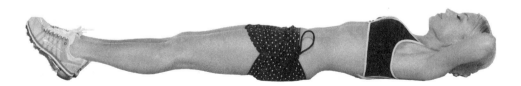

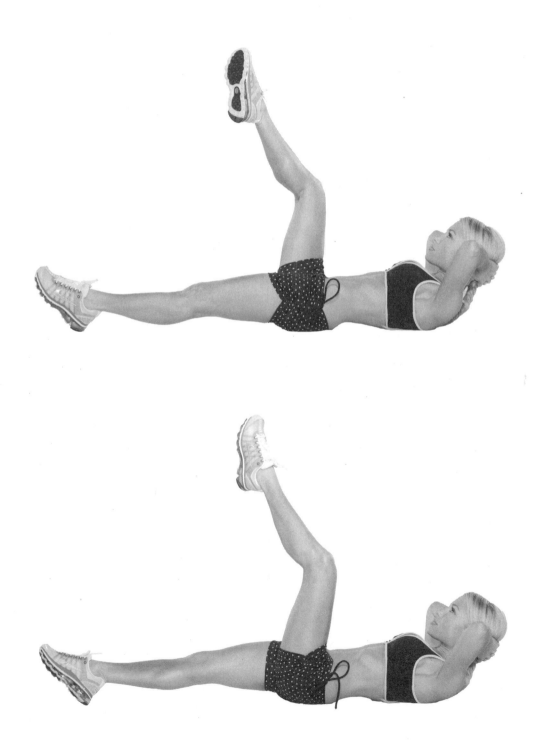

Move #10: Cross Leg Crunches

The challenge is to do this move without lifting your butt cheek off the floor while you're crunching and crossing. This action will encourage the very important bolting in your hip flexors.

Stance: Lie on your back with your feet spread mat distance apart. Hands are behind your head. Toes are pointed.

Action: As you crunch up by lifting your head and shoulders, move your right leg over your left leg, crossing at the ankle (remember to keep your butt on the floor). As you relax back, extend your leg back to center. Crunch up, and cross your left leg over your right leg, then relax and extend.

Flow: Continue crunching and crossing, right over left, and then left over right.

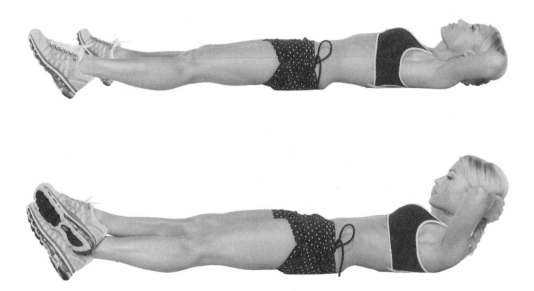

Move #11: Crunch with Leg Tuck and Extend

The last crunch of the series. The cross-vector here happens at the point at which your legs carry energy toward your feet and beyond, and your upper body reaches in the opposite direction.

Stance: Begin on your back with your legs together and extended. Raise your legs slightly off the ground. Arms are behind your head.

Action: Crunch up with your knees while lifting your head and shoulders toward your chest, then extend your legs out in the air and hold for one second. Crunch up, knees to your head, and extend out, keeping your legs together.

Flow: Continue crunching, head to knees, and extending and holding.

A beginner's version of this move is to do your crunch and tuck—then, when you extend, let your feet come down on the ground. But I really don't want you to become handicapped more than you need to be. If over the first few days you find yourself dropping your feet to the floor a few times, that's fine. The next baby step would be to crunch up and drop just one leg at a time. That way you're at least strengthening your abs and hip flexors so your muscles can learn to hold the weight of the legs.

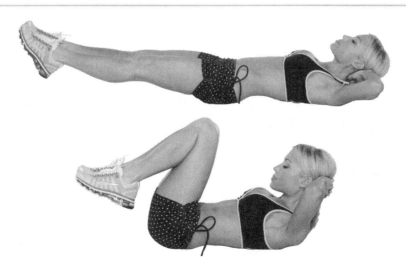

Move #12: Connection Push-Up

This variation on the classic push-up helps connect all your muscles together. By the time you're doing Sequence 3, you're really going to be challenged by connecting exercises. At this stage, I'm giving you the chance to strengthen and wake up all the parts of your body that will support you so you can do the more advanced work.

Stance: Get into a classic push-up position. Adjust your feet so that they're wider than the mat, about three feet apart.

Action: Touch your right knee to the ground. Then straighten it back out. Repeat. The cross-vector happens when you press back so the heel stretches the hamstring, and your upper body reaches forward toward the opposite side of the room.

Flow: Continue touching the knee to the ground and then straightening the leg for ten reps; repeat on the left side. After a full set, touch both knees down for ten reps.

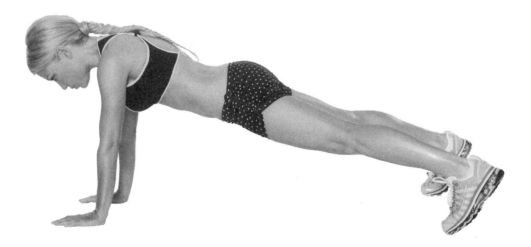

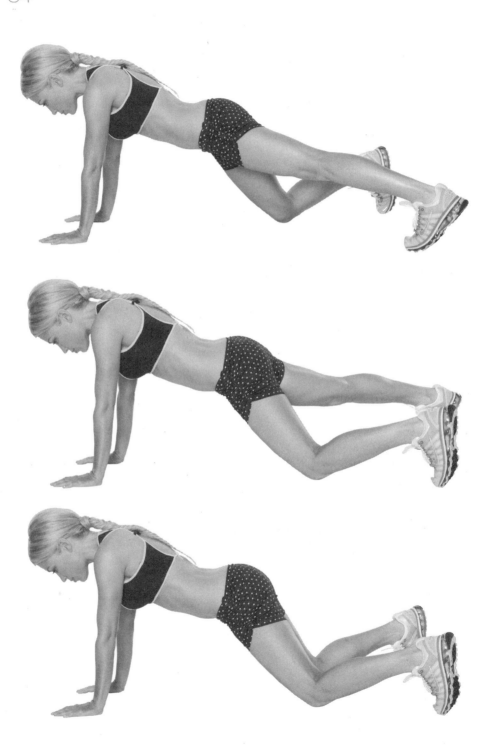

Move #13: Arm Reach

You're not going to use weights to make your arms fabulous and teeny tiny and beautiful. Instead, you're going to use the cross-vectors that you can activate by really reaching and pulling.

Stance: Kneel, or sit with your legs crossed; either way, keep your spine straight. Stretch your arms out to the sides, and turn your palms to face the front of the room.

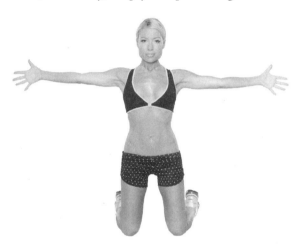

Action: Bend your elbows slightly so that the palms face up. Then reach your arms apart from each other, palms facing front again. Really reach through as actively as you can, waking up all your muscles and activating the cross-vectors.

Picture someone standing on each side of you, pulling your arms, someone else pulling your head up (gently), and a third person pressing down on your shoulders. You have to create that energy yourself. When you reach your arms out to the side, cross-vectors occur in a couple of places. One is located across your back, where your arms stretch in opposite directions. The other is between your ears and your shoulders: You want to create as much space in your neck as possible, so your head reaches up, toward the ceiling, and your shoulders reach down your back.

Flow: Reach and then bend, reach and then bend.

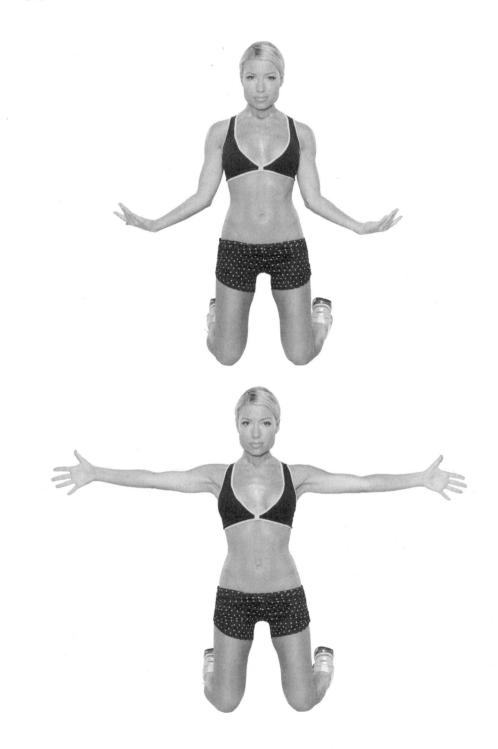

Move #14: Alternate Arm Hit

This arm exercise incorporates the same principles as the arm reach, with some additions.

Stance: Kneel, or sit with your legs crossed, spine straight. Stretch your arms out to the sides. Turn your palms to face the front of the room. Bend your elbows slightly.

Action: Reach the energy of your arm to the right while your torso pulls in the opposite direction (there's your cross-vector). Reach as if there's a basketball bouncing just out of reach and in front of you, and you're going to smack it away. Keep your arms straight and then flick through the wrist.

Flow: Reach and smack to the right, shifting toward the right at your waist, and then do the same thing to the left.

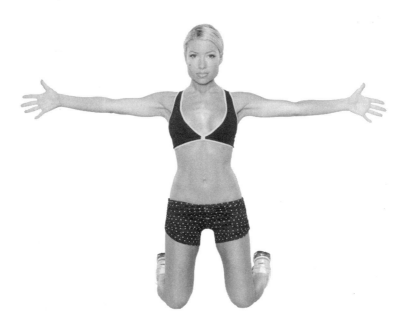

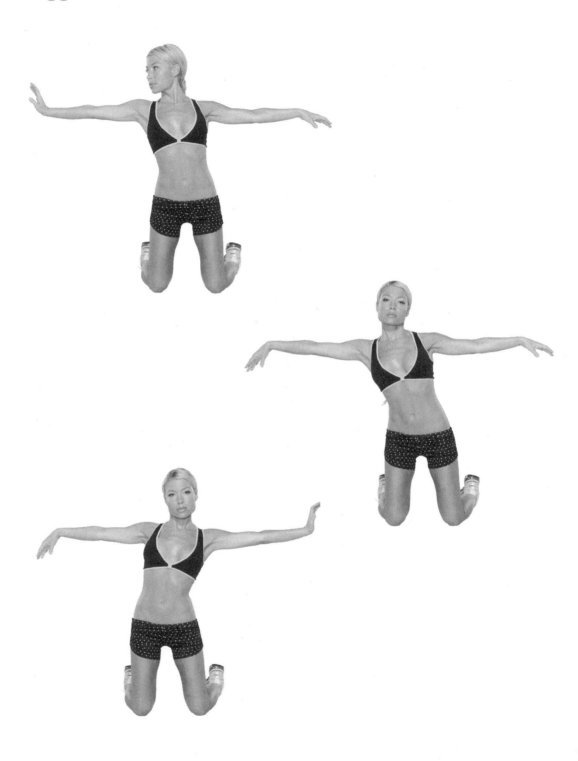

Move #15: Basketball Palm Rotation

If you don't reach actively, if you're just holding your arms like deadweight, you're going to bulk up and develop neck issues. It isn't proper form. So head up, shoulders down, arms out to the sides, really reaching.

Stance: Kneel, or sit with your legs crossed, keeping your spine straight. Stretch your arms out to the sides. Turn your palms to the ceiling, fingers curled up slightly, like you're holding two basketballs.

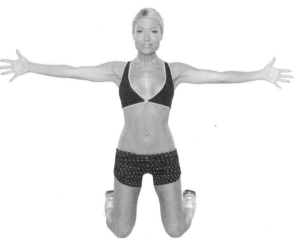

Action: Gripping those imaginary basketballs, rotate your hands from the shoulders, rolling them over so your thumbs move toward the front of the room, as if you're holding the basketballs from the top.

Flow: Move your arms around and over, and back. Around and over, and back, like you're carving C's in the air with your arms.

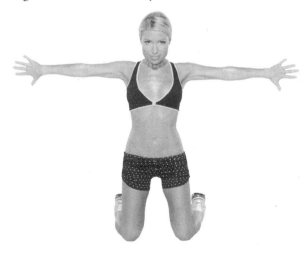

Move #16: Low W High V Arm Reach

When you reach up, really try to touch the ceiling. When you pull down into the W, don't just drop your arms—make sure all the muscles are active and involved.

Stance: Kneel, or sit with your legs crossed and your spine straight. Stretch your arms out to the sides. Palms face front.

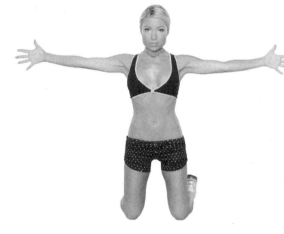

Action: Bend your elbows toward your hips, palms facing up so that you're making a W with your upper body. Now raise your arms up toward the ceiling in a V for Victory.

Flow: Move smoothly from W to V, keeping all your arm muscles engaged, and creating a cross-vector by really reaching your arms away from each other as you stretch for the sky.

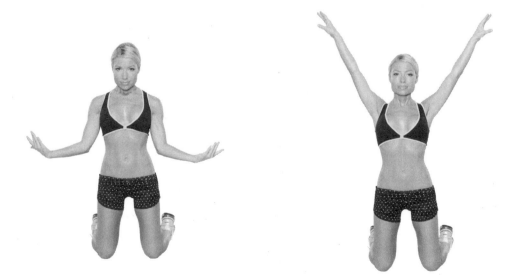

Sequence 2: Days 11–20

You've made it to the second sequence, and while your body has become accustomed to the moves you were doing over the first ten days, things are about to change. You can expect to feel exhausted at the end of the first two days in the same way that you did in the first sequence, as I push you a little further and your body learns some new lessons.

The second sequence is aimed at improving your connection with your brain. There is so much power in your brain and its relationship to the muscles. When your brain is challenged, you use your muscles in a different way. When your balance is challenged, you use your muscles in a different way. My Method uses the brain to teach the muscles to contract and react, and engage more fully based on the circumstances in which you hold and move your body.

For the second ten days, days 11 through 20, I've incorporated a chair into the workout. As we talked about earlier, you'll need a sturdy kitchen chair with a strong back: something that you won't be afraid will topple while you do moves that have you step up on the seat or balance with one hand on the chair. You're going to learn to become aware of your proprioception—feeling where your body is in space—and how your muscles are working. It's an understanding of your place in the world based on your muscles instead of on your eyes or ears. The mirrors let you use your exteroceptive sense—seeing—to understand how your body is moving. But eventually your proprioceptive abilities will improve and you will really be able to perform the moves.

Even though you're still working at a basic level—you aren't up on a balance beam or a trapeze, you're on a chair, close to the ground—you'll have to engage a new type of balance and awareness.

The second ten days is about training the brain to connect with the body so you can trigger your accessory muscles on a new level.

So let's get started.

Move #17: Straight Leg Knee Pull

Precision is what makes perfection possible. When you reach your leg back, make sure that your foot is at least an inch above your hip.

Stance: Stand behind the chair with your arms straight out in front of you, hands placed on the back of the chair.

Action: Lean forward, bending your elbows, and raise your right leg behind you with your hip slightly open, foot pointed to the back of the room. Your leg and your torso are in one long line. Pull your knee forward toward your armpit, keeping your hip open and keeping the knee raised slightly higher than your foot. Then extend it back.

> Engage the cross-vector by reaching your right shoulder forward as the foot reaches behind.

Flow: Your leg contracts forward, and then it extends and expands out. Pull the knee forward, and extend it back. Pull and extend.

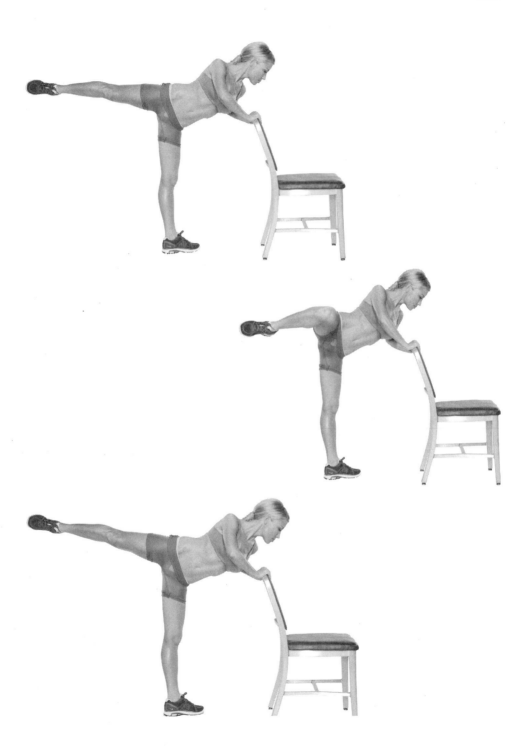

Move #18: Straight Leg Side and Behind with Pulse

You've already set the mark for how high you can raise your leg behind you. Now is not the time to compromise. Maintain the integrity.

Stance: Stand behind the chair with your arms straight out in front of you, hands placed on the back of the chair.

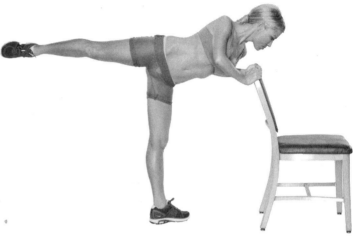

Action: Raise your right leg behind you as you did in the last move, right hip slightly open to the side, but instead of pulling your knee toward your armpit, you're going to swing your leg to the right at hip height until it's straight out to the right side, with your right knee and toes pointing forward. Then swing it back behind you and lift it up, slightly higher than straight behind you, with a little pulse.

Flow: Side, behind, lift. Side, behind, lift.

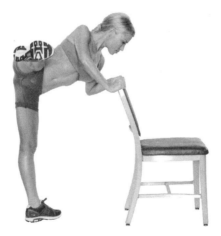

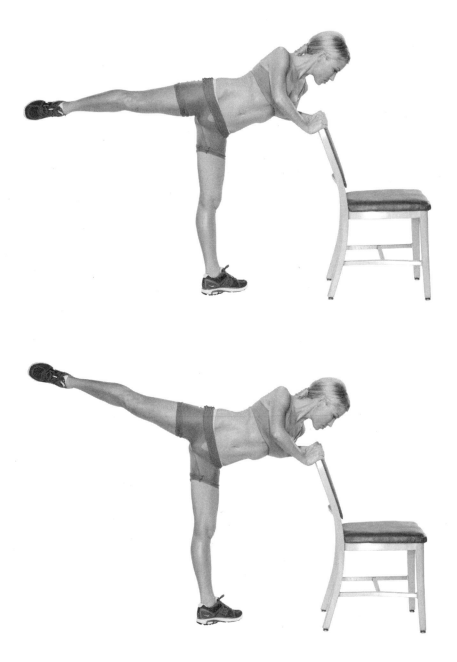

Move #19: Hand on Ground, Leg Lifts and Straightens

This is where you really start to connect all the muscles together.

Stance: Kneel on the seat of the chair with your left side next to the back of the chair, and place your left hand on the floor.

> Holding your arm down on the ground is going to become challenging. That's good. You're going to really work through that.

Action: Raise your right leg, knee bent at a right angle, up to the side. Then return it to neutral (raised in the air, with knee still bent) and extend it at an upward diagonal behind you, to the left. The hand on the ground reaches down into the ground to stabilize you while your right foot reaches way up and to the left, activating the cross-vectors of force. Bring the leg back in, bending your knee at a right angle.

Flow: Knee comes down, lift to the side, back in, and extend it out.

> Make sure that you hit your mark. If you don't have your *ta-da!* moment, where your leg reaches all the way up, then you haven't done your job right.

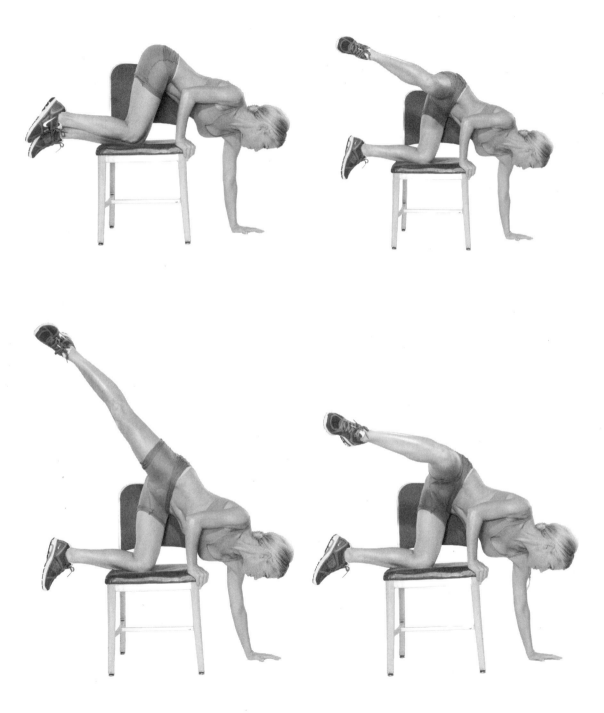

Move #20: Step Up Attitude Lift

Stepping up on a chair can be somewhat challenging, so make sure you have a nice, sturdy chair.

Stance: Place your left foot on the seat of the chair (from the front).

Action: You're going to step up, balance yourself with your hands on the back of the chair for support, and then reach your leg up as high as you can in a turned-out attitude position, knee slightly bent, toes pointed to the ceiling. Bring the leg back down, touch the ground for a split second, and then launch right back up.

Flow: Launch up, attitude, and down. Up, attitude, and down.

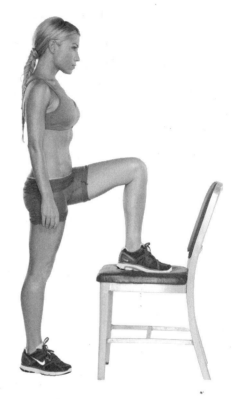

You don't want to open up the hip of the leg that's kicking in this one. In order to activate the cross-vector, when your right foot is reaching up in an attitude, your right hip is reaching to the ground. Two directions at once.

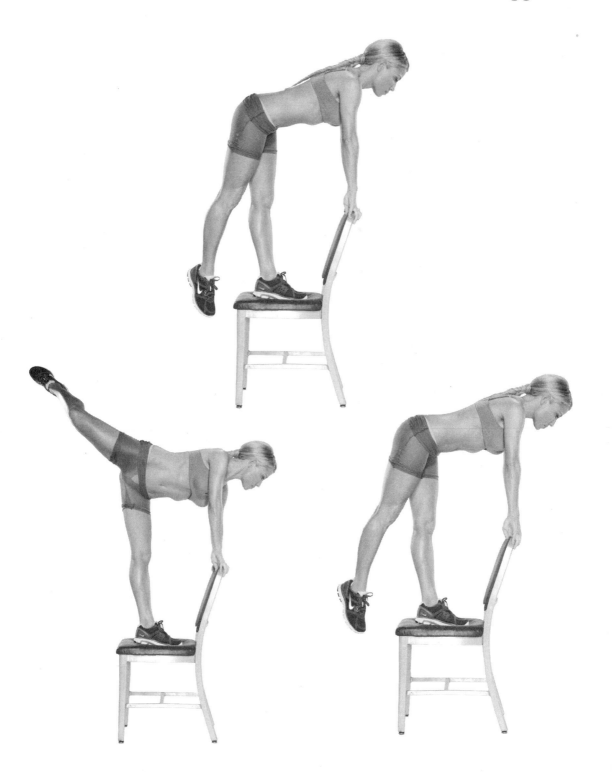

Move #21: Kneeling Diagonal Knee Touch with Pulse

This move uses a leg position you'll remember from the first sequence, but you'll be incorporating it in a new way. The seat of the chair reminds you to stay honest and keep your leg above hip height.

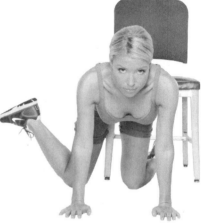

Stance: Get on your hands and knees in front of the chair. Your left foot rests under the chair's seat. Your right knee is bent in an inverted position, to the right. Knees together. Right toe is out.

Action: Lift your leg with a turned-in knee, moving the foot back, slightly up and to the right of the chair, leg straight. Pulse up to the ceiling, then swing the leg to the side and back to neutral (knees down and together, foot to the right).

Flow: Lift, pulse, and return. Lift, pulse, and return.

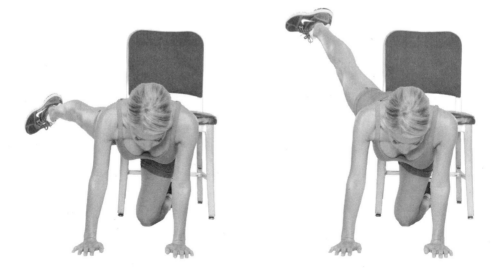

Move #22: Diagonal Tuck and Sweep

You'll be lifting your leg behind you to the left and right of the chair, using the chair as a point of reference for your range of motion.

Stance: Get on your hands and knees in front of the chair, feet just in front of and even with the chair's legs.

Action: Extend your right leg behind you to the right of the chair. Then tuck it in, keeping your weight forward on your hands so you can extend the same leg behind you to the left side, on the other side of the chair.

Flow: Maintain the integrity of the severe diagonal on both sides of the chair. Right side, left side. Right side, left side.

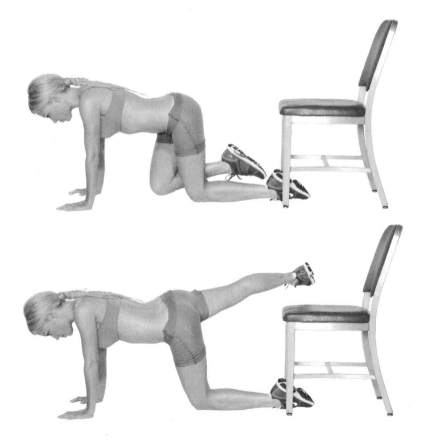

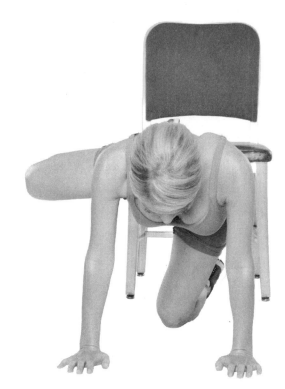

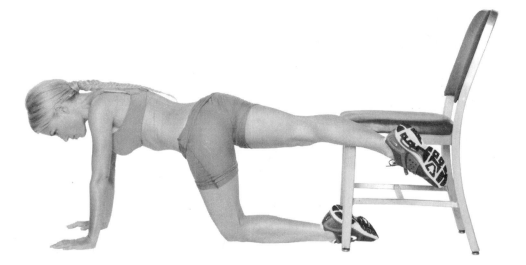

Move #23: Side Run Scissor Split

For this final leg exercise, you don't need to use the chair. Think of this move as a combination of a run, with bent knees, and a scissor kick with straight legs.

Stance: Lie on your left side with your left arm supporting yourself. Both knees are slightly bent.

Action: Tuck your right knee in toward your chest. Then extend your left leg forward, and your right leg behind, straightening both legs as you extend them forward and back. As the top leg swings back, it moves with a bend in the knee and then straightens at the resolution. Meanwhile, the bottom leg is straightening and extending forward.

Reach your right hip forward as your right foot reaches back to activate the cross-vectors.

Flow: Tuck the top leg forward, extend it back to a straight leg. Meanwhile, extend your bent bottom leg forward and straighten. Then the top leg tucks forward again and the bottom leg bends to return to neutral (bent position). Tuck, extend, return.

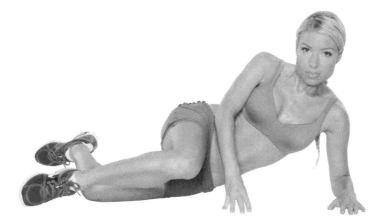

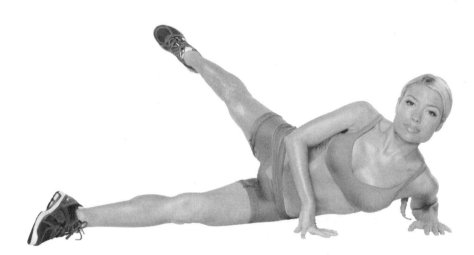

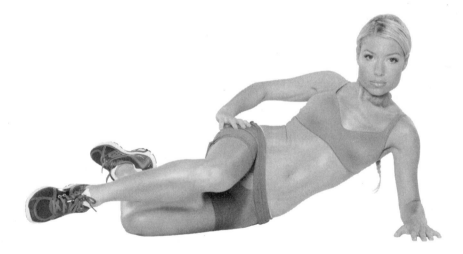

Move #24: Straight Leg Crunches with Single Arm Reach

You're going to use the Straight Leg Crunches again—but this time, you'll reach one arm at a time up toward the ceiling. Reaching with just one arm engages the ab muscles in a completely different way.

Stance: Lie on your back, legs extended straight in front of you, toes pointing to the front of the room. Keep your right hand behind your head; you aren't quite ready to crunch without supporting your neck.

Action: Crunch up, and reach with your left hand, supporting the neck with your right hand. Then switch. Crunch up, and reach with your right hand, supporting the neck with your left.

As you reach your right arm up, your left shoulder should fight back for the ground. When you reach the left arm up, the right shoulder should fight to stay on the ground. The key to engaging the cross-vector forces is that you really, really reach.

Flow: Crunch and reach left. Crunch and reach right.

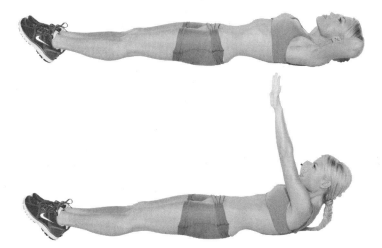

Move #25: Tuck Crunch with Diagonal Leg Extension

This is a really important one. It's going to be challenging. That's why, during the first ten-day sequence, I asked you to make sure that when you did the Crunch with Leg Tuck and Extend you didn't just drop your legs down. Now you need to be able to maintain that position, only at a whole different level.

Stance: Lie on your back, legs extended straight in front of you, toes pointing to the front of the room. Place your hands behind your head.

Action: Crunch up while you tuck your legs in, and then extend your legs out. Lift your right leg up and twist slightly toward the left. Keep your left leg slightly off the floor. Tuck in, then lift your left leg up and twist slightly to the right as you extend.

Good form on this sequence is important. Most women don't ever get the lower abs that they want because they work them in a flat way. You need to twist your muscles and challenge them on different levels and planes. Especially if you've had children, you've got to break up the scar tissue. You have to learn to connect those muscles and knit them in a different way. As women, our bodies want to pouch out in our lower abs. To keep that area nice and flat, we have to really work them in an intelligent way.

If you need to modify this move, when you tuck in, lay your bottom leg on the ground. Keep the top leg in position. This way, when you're ready to lift the bottom one, you can.

Flow: Maintain the crunch throughout, supporting your head with your arms. Tuck your legs in, then extend and twist. Tuck, extend and twist, switching sides each time.

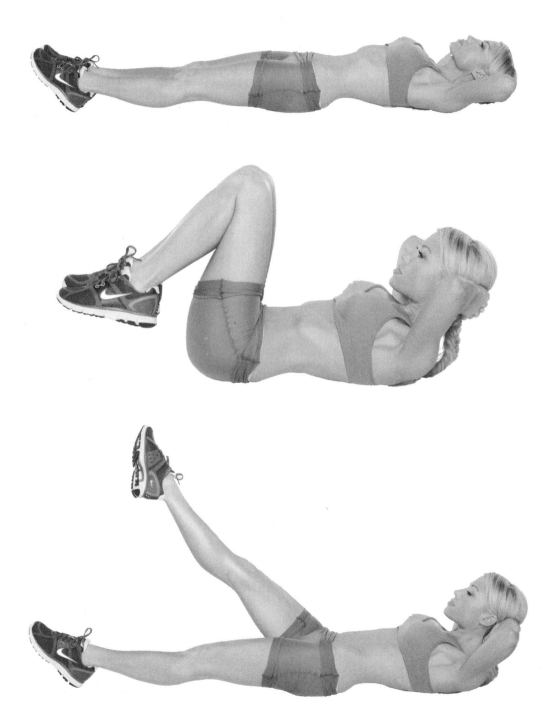

Move #26: Legs Apart Diagonal Reach

Breathe easy...with this move, you'll get to keep your legs down.

Stance: Lie on your back, legs apart in a V wider than your mat. Toes point to the front of the room. Hands behind your head.

Action: Crunch up and reach your right arm down your right leg on a diagonal and beyond. I need this to be a big reach. Relax back. Then crunch up and reach your right arm toward the ceiling.

> Keep supporting your head and neck with the arm that isn't reaching.

Flow: Alternate crunches and arm movements: Crunch with your right arm reaching down your right leg, crunch with your right arm reaching up to the ceiling. Repeat all your reps on the right side. Then repeat on the left side.

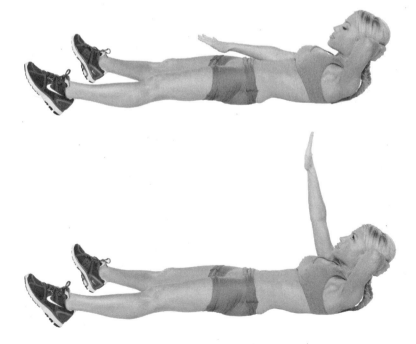

Move #27: Double Pike with Single Leg Straight Drop

Pikes are really important for your ab work, so make sure to try your hardest here to do the action correctly.

Stance: Lie on your back, legs together and straight. Toes point to the front of the room.

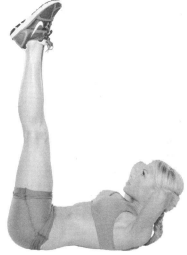

Action: Keeping your legs together, lift them to ninety degrees. Place your hands behind your head. When your legs are extending straight toward the ceiling, knees straight, you're going to crunch. Bend your left knee and then lower your straight right leg down, hovering two inches above the ground. Then bring your right leg back up to ninety degrees and straighten your left leg. Repeat, alternating sides.

Flow: Crunch and raise both legs. Bend your left knee, sweep your straight right leg down, and hover. Raise your right leg and straighten your left leg. Bend your right leg, sweep your straight left leg down, and hover. Repeat. Alternate sides as you do your reps.

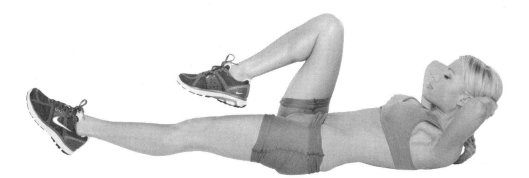

Move #28: Push-Up Diagonal Leg Lift

This alternative to the classic push-up challenges the whole body. Keep your arms straight throughout this move.

Stance: Begin in push-up position, with your legs slightly wider than shoulder width apart. Weight is evenly distributed between your hands and feet; abs are pulled in. This will be your neutral position.

Action: Keeping your arms straight, drop your hips to the ground. Pass through neutral and lift your right leg in attitude, then lift it up behind you, straightening the leg and crossing it over your left hip toward the ceiling. Move back through neutral and drop your hips to the ground again, arms straight. Now switch sides, raising your hips and then your left leg in the attitude position, and then lifting the left leg behind you to the ceiling.

Finding the cross-vectors: When you drop your hips, lift your chest toward the ceiling. As you coil your lower abdominals back up to a plank position, your right hip is going to reach in the opposite direction of your right heel.

Flow: Hips to the ground, then back up as your right leg sweeps up in attitude position to raise, straighten, and lift behind you up toward the ceiling, crossing the midline slightly. Hips to the ground, then back up as your left leg sweeps up in attitude position to raise, straighten, and lift behind you up toward the ceiling.

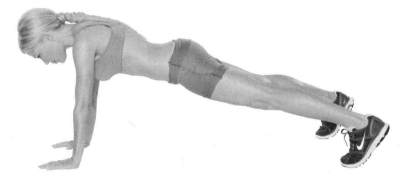

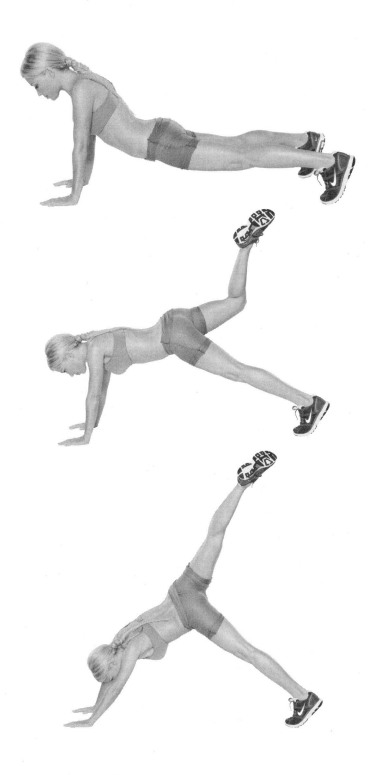

Move #29: Hit Hit Double Hit

For the second sequence, you're going to stand for the arm exercises. The first one is going to be the same hitting motion as the Alternate Arm Hit from Sequence 1, but this time you're gonna hit with more rhythm: Hit, hit, and double hit.

Stance: Stand tall with your spine straight. Stretch your arms out to the sides actively, turning your palms to face the front of the room. Bend your elbows slightly.

Action: Reach the energy of your arm to the right, while your torso pulls in the opposite direction (that's what's going to engage your cross-vector). Reach like there's a basketball bouncing just out of reach and in front of you, and you're going to smack it away. Keep your arms straight and then flick through the wrist. That's the hit. When you do your double hit, you're going to smack to the ground, palm down, and then back to the front of the room.

Flow: Reach and smack front to the right, reach and smack front to the left, reach and smack down to the right, front to the right. Reach and smack front to the left, reach and smack front to the right, reach and smack down to the left, front to the left. Single hit, single hit, double hit. Hit, hit, double hit.

Make sure to lean your hips to the left when you smack to the right, and vice versa.

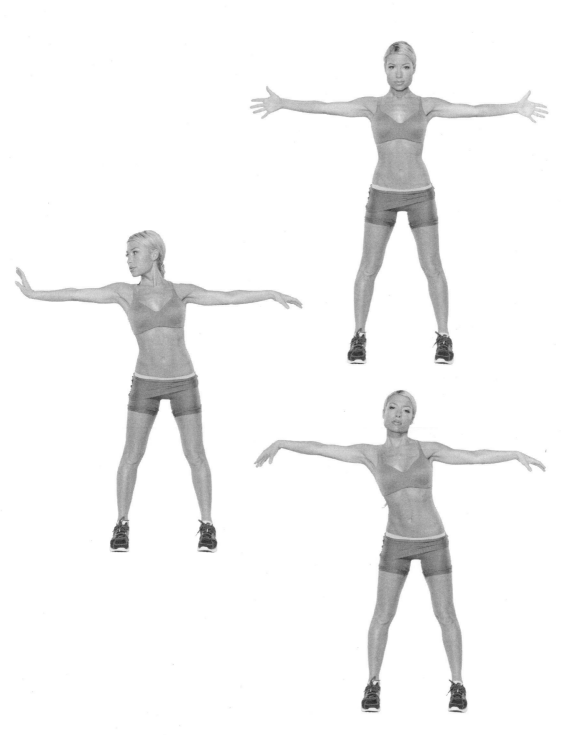

Move #30: Thumbs Up Thumbs Down Lift

Maintain the integrity throughout this movement, moving smoothly and with purpose.

Stance: Stand tall with your feet shoulder width apart, arms reaching to the sides. Palms face the front of the room (thumbs point to the ceiling).

Action: Lift your arms to higher than shoulder height, palms facing front, thumbs up. Then twist your arms from the shoulder so that your palms face back and your thumbs are down. Your arms should be straight and active the whole time.

Flow: Palms front, thumbs up. Palms back, thumbs down.

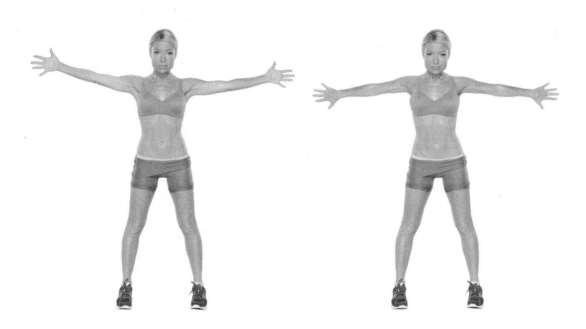

Move #31: Straight Arm Back with Hits

The cross-vector here comes from reaching your shoulder forward as your wrist and arm reach behind you, as if you're trying to hit someone behind you from a really awkward position.

Stance: Stand tall on your mat, feet a little wider than shoulder width apart. Place your left hand on your hip and extend your right arm, thumb down, palm open to the back of the room.

Action: Swing your right arm back at shoulder level, and return the arm to its starting position. Then hit back higher, way above your head, as if you're reaching back and hitting someone much taller than you. Your hand must reach behind your shoulder each time—remember to hit from the wrist. This action is a lot easier when you're just hitting back, so maintain the integrity as you hit back and up.

Flow: Hit back low, hit back high. Hit back low, hit back high. Do all your reps on the right side, then all your reps on the left.

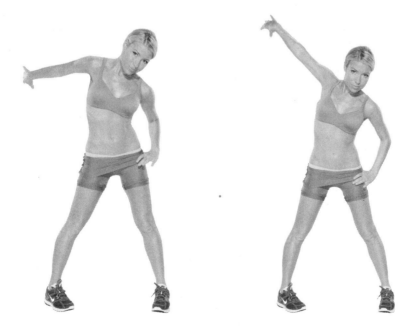

Move #32: W Arm Pull-Down and Press

Almost done for the day!

Stance: Stand tall on your mat, feet a little wider than shoulder width apart. Your left hand is on your hip. Your right hand is raised straight up in the air a few inches to the right side, as if in a one-armed V for victory, palm facing in toward your body.

Action: Using your right elbow to lead the motion, pull your arm down to your side so that instead of half a V shape, it's making half a W shape. Raise your arm back up, rotate the palm and press your arm straight down to your side, then back up again into your half V.

Flow: W-arm pull, rotate, straight arm palm press down. Up and down W. Up and down press. When you have completed both sides, you will do a set of reps moving both arms together, from full V position down to W, up to V and down with the straight arm press on both sides. Do all your reps on your right side, then on your left side, then with both arms.

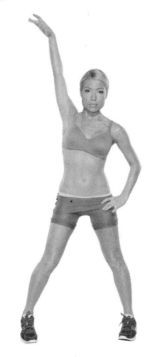

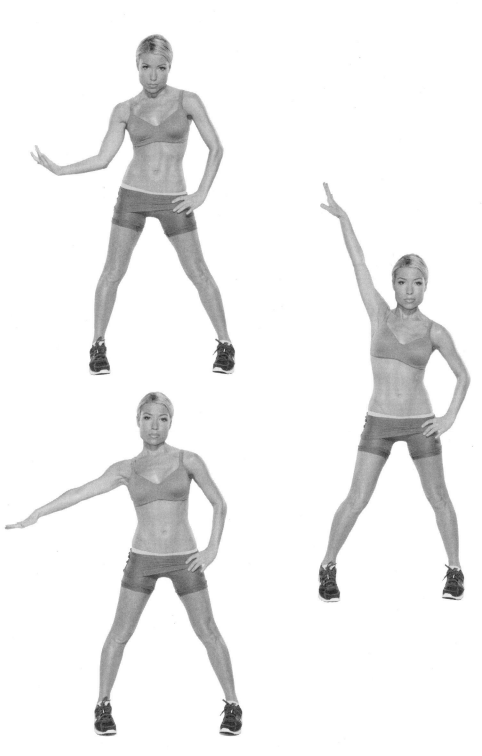

Sequence 3: Days 21-30

With this third ten-day sequence, we're really going to challenge the body on a lot of different levels. The chair is back, but we're not using it as a balancing prop. We're using it to engage our muscles in a new way, and the hand positioning on the chair is very, very important. Whether or not you think you need help balancing, pay attention to the hand placement. Just the tactile sense of it either triggers or relaxes a muscle that you need to engage.

This is an exciting part of the 30-Day Method. It is when you'll begin to really see your results. It's when unbelievable things start happening. And this is why: You're pushing yourself to a whole other level of performance.

During the third ten days, the exercises are designed to go after the places in the body where you can bolt your muscles. I'm talking about the "miracle" areas that make sure the lower abs are flat, or that the hips don't bulge, or that your bottom stays perfectly lifted. The places that eradicate back fat and underarm sag.

Usually, when you have problem areas, the proposed fitness solution is to attack the problem directly. For instance, have an issue with your lower abs? Traditional programs offer ab exercises that target the obvious muscles—your abs—but the problem doesn't go away. With my Method, while the abs themselves get a workout, I am also targeting the *effective* muscles instead of just the *obvious* ones. I focus on the muscles that are next to the problem areas as well as the problem areas themselves. By following your lines to where the muscles collect, I can create a contraction to encourage the kind of effective change that will make an obvious difference.

At this level, you really need to understand the depth of power your brain has in controlling your personal results levels. Because if you're here but you aren't performing, if you're distracted instead of focused, if you're just going from point A to point B without any through-line of energy and thought, your results are going to occur very slowly. But if you really connect, and you really feel the movements, and you use your power—if you can become like an animal, using your instincts instead of your rational brain—like a jaguar chasing its prey—you're going to get the adrenaline rush. And you're going to get the results.

Move #33: Foot Front Diagonal Attitude Back

The cross-vector happens right away, when you lift your knee. The knee needs to be lifted as high as it can.

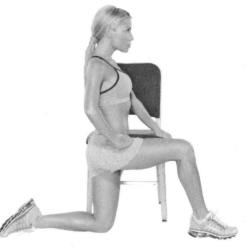

Stance: Kneel at the front of the chair, facing sideways. Place your right foot in front of you, knee bent to ninety degrees. Your left hand is on the seat of the chair.

Action: Lift your knee up, and sweep it to the side and back into an attitude (bent to ninety degrees). Engage your glute muscles, and lift your knee. As you're rotating your knee to the side, your hip flexor and your right hip will come forward as part of the attitude, and the attitude is also lifting up toward the ceiling. Your knee remains bent slightly the whole time. Return to starting position.

Flow: Lift and sweep and lift to the back, leg still in attitude position, and return. Lift and sweep and lift and return.

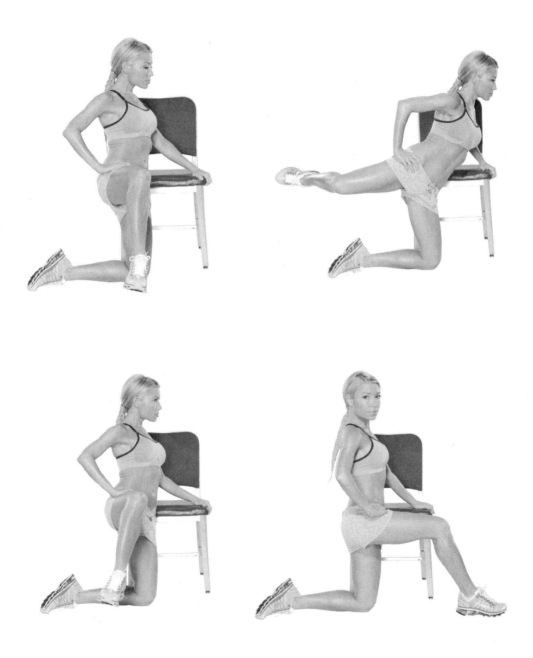

Move #34: Three Pulse Attitude Climbing Kick

The cross-vector here happens when your right shoulder reaches forward in the direction opposite your foot. Pay attention to those little things. They really matter.

Stance: Kneel in front of the chair, with your right leg bent at a right angle, right foot on the floor. Your left hand is on the seat of the chair for balance. Right hand on your hip.

Action: Raise your right leg to the back, keeping the knee slightly bent in a turned-out attitude position. Then straighten that leg slightly below your right hip. Pulse the kick higher, then pulse it as high as you can. The pulses will climb in the air, and then the leg returns to hip height to begin the three-pulse cycle again. Return to starting position at the end of each cycle. Remember, shoulder moves forward as leg moves back.

Flow: Lower, high, and up. Lower, high, and up.

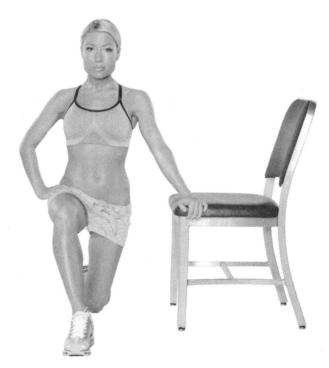

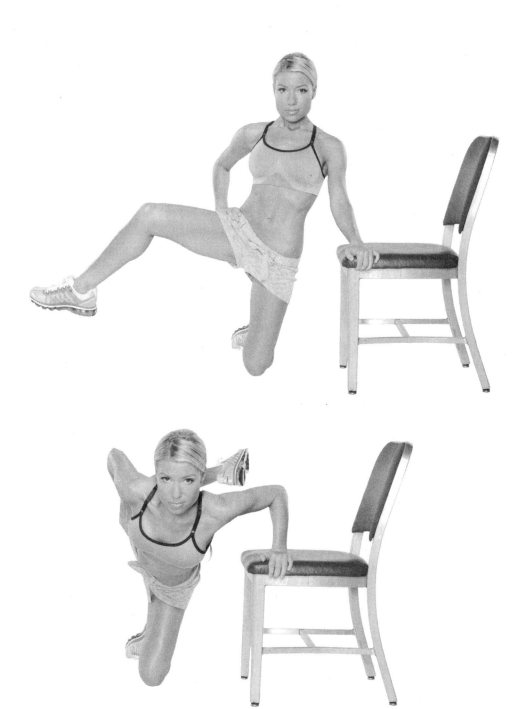

Move #35: Push-Up with One Hand on Chair and Diagonal Leg Tuck

This is for your abs, arms, butt…we're really knitting everything together now.

Stance: Get into push-up position in front of the chair, left side next to the chair. Your feet are spread wider than your shoulders. Place your left hand on the seat of the chair and keep your right hand in a push-up position on the ground.

Action: Bring your right knee in, and then extend it back and up on a diagonal. Bring it in, and then extend it back again. The challenge of the cross-vector will be in your left hip, stabilizing and pulling down to the ground, as your right leg moves diagonally back.

> You're going to really feel this in your oblique muscles (your lower abs). That's what's going to engage and stabilize you. After the first twenty days of your kick start, your muscles will have really woken up, so you'll feel this in a new way, and that's what's exciting.

Flow: Knee in and extend back. Knee in and extend back.

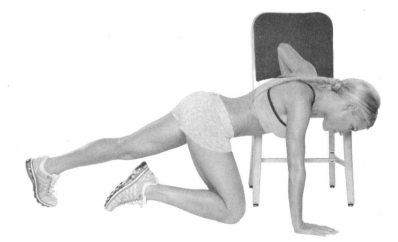

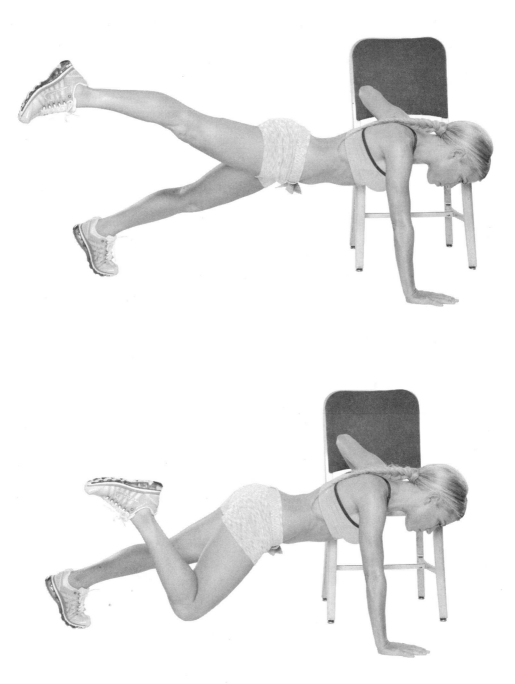

Move #36: Inner Thigh Pull with Hands on Chair

This move targets the inner thighs. The cross-vector is in the hips.

Stance: Sit at the edge of the chair with your hands holding the chair by your butt, legs bent in front of you. Slip your butt off the chair so your straight arms and bent legs are holding you up, almost as if you're still sitting.

Action: Keep your hands on the base of the chair, and extend your right leg out to the right side, straightening it; then pull it back across your body, bending at the knee as if you're about to cross your legs.

> The cross-vector, again, is in the hips. As your foot goes out to the side, the right hip should be reaching forward. You'll also be sinking into your left hip.

Flow: Keeping yourself up on your arms, extend, straighten, and cross your leg. Extend, straighten, and cross.

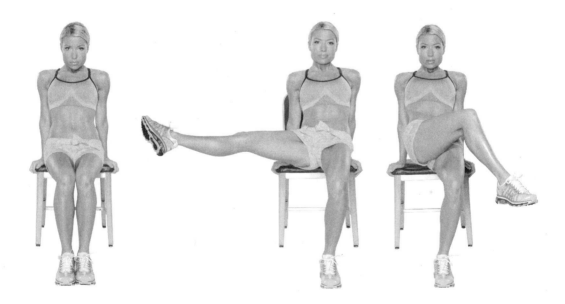

Move #37: Downward Dog Split with Side Sweep

If you've ever done yoga, this move will feel familiar to you: It utilizes many of the same principles as Downward Dog. Use the back of the chair as a guide to keep your leg raised as high as you can.

Stance: Begin in Downward Dog stance to the left of your chair. (The chair should be on your right.) Both hands on the floor, shoulder distance apart, and both feet on the floor, hips high in the air.

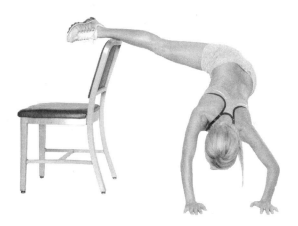

Action: Raise your right leg high in the air so you're basically doing a Downward Dog split, creating a nice long line from your right arm up through your leg. Sweep your raised leg down, knee facing forward, so it just barely skims the top of the back of your chair, and then extend it back up behind you. When your leg is raised up as high as possible behind you, your arms are pushing back so they are in a diagonal line from the floor. When your leg is out to your side, you are pushing forward onto your arms, so your arms are straight.

The cross-vector is, again, in the hips. As your leg goes back, your hip is coming forward. As your leg sweeps to the side, you have to keep your hips straight.

Flow: Raise the leg, then sweep it down to the side, then sweep it back up. Raise it, then sweep it.

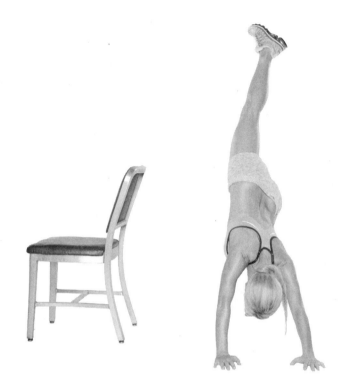

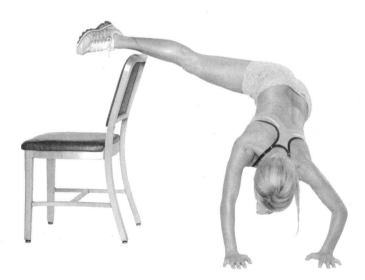

Move #38: Knee on Chair, Lift Diagonal and Back

Don't rely on momentum here to move your leg—I want you to really use your muscles.

Stance: Get on your hands and knees slightly in front of the chair with your right side to the chair's seat. Raise your right leg to the side and set it on the seat, still bent, with the inside of your knee resting on the chair.

Action: Lift your leg up, knee bent, and then straighten the leg to the side so that the foot extends above the back of the chair. With this move, your left hip will go forward, your right leg will reach at an upward diagonal, and you're going to sink into your left elbow. Return to neutral. (See the box below.)

> Each time you return to neutral, you're going to put all the weight of your leg back down on the chair. I want you to really set it down so you have to reengage it every time.

Flow: Lift your leg and straighten it, then return to bent position.

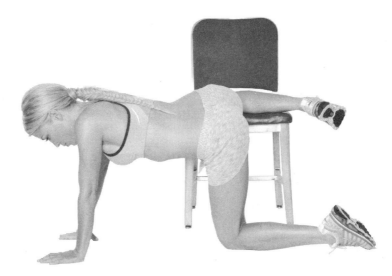

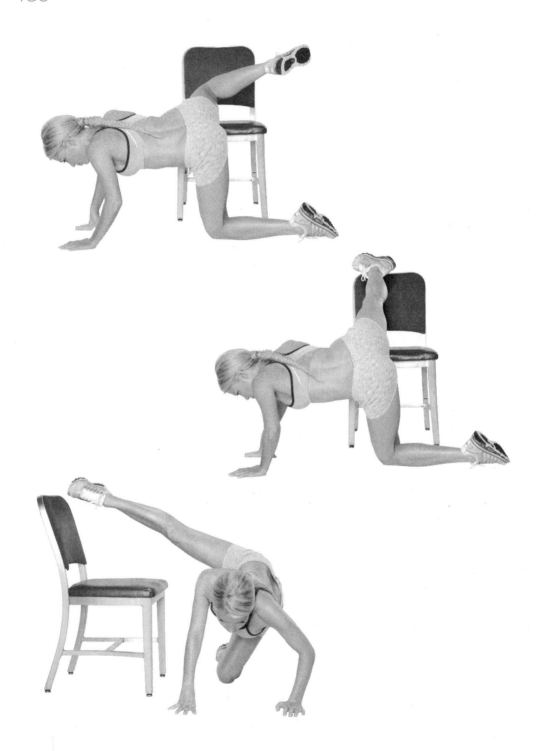

Move #39: Hand to Chair, Hand to Ground, High Back Kick

A great one for your butt—make sure you kick that leg up as high as it will go behind you.

Stance: Stand so the chair is on your right. Lift your right leg and place your right foot on the seat, toes pointing to the right. Hands are on your hips.

Action: Lift your right knee up and sweep it back. As you do this, lean forward: Your right hand goes to the chair and your left hand reaches for the ground. Kick the leg up as high as you can and then return it to the chair.

Flow: Lift and lean, kick as high as you can. Lift and lean, kick as high as you can.

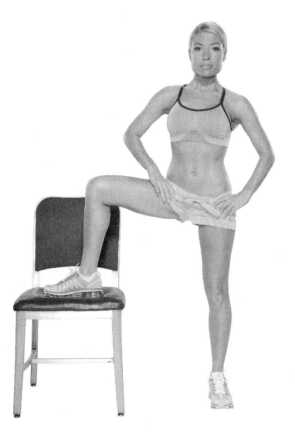

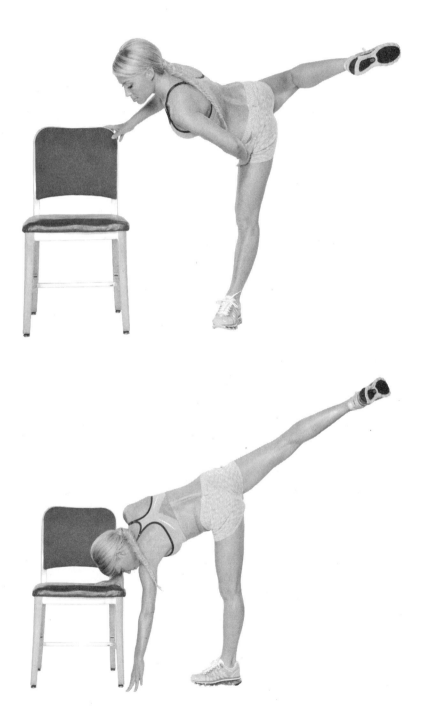

Move #40: Bent Knee to Back Kick Swivel, with Floor Touch

This one requires a bit of swivel...remember to stay engaged!

Stance: Stand to the left side of the chair (so it's on your right). Place your right leg on the seat, knee bent. Hands are on your hips.

Action: Swivel on your left foot so that you are facing the chair. Your right leg swings up and back, kicking through bent knee. Meanwhile, your right hand comes to the seat of the chair, and your left hand touches the floor. Then you'll stand again, swiveling back on your foot, raised leg returning to its bent-knee position on the chair.

Flow: Raise the leg and touch the floor and the chair, then swivel, stand, and return to neutral (foot on chair). Repeat.

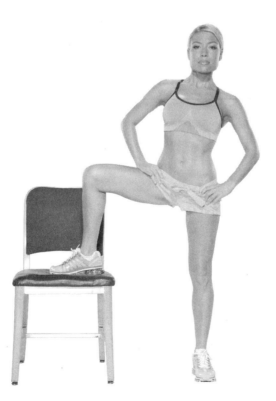

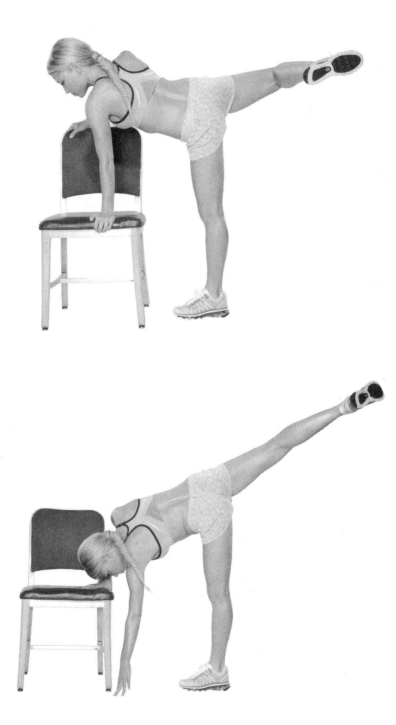

Move #41: Bent Tuck with Attitude Lift and Sweep

Keep your abs engaged during this move as you tuck, stand and lift, and rotate your leg.

Stance: Stand facing the left side of the chair, legs together. Place your hands on the seat of the chair. You will be in a tucked position.

Action: Lift up on the balls of your feet, and then squat down to the ground. Your hands are still on the chair in position, and you are still on the balls of your feet. Use your arms to bring you up to straight legs, maintaining their position on the chair. With legs straight, lift your right leg back in attitude and sweep it around behind you, crossing the midline as you straighten. Then return the leg to attitude and bring it back to neutral, squatting back on the ground.

Flow: From a squat, straighten your legs, hands on chair. Lift your leg in attitude, sweep to the back and straighten, then return to an attitude and back to neutral.

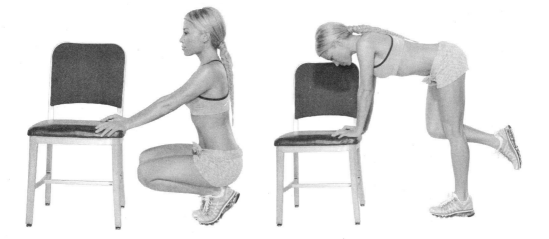

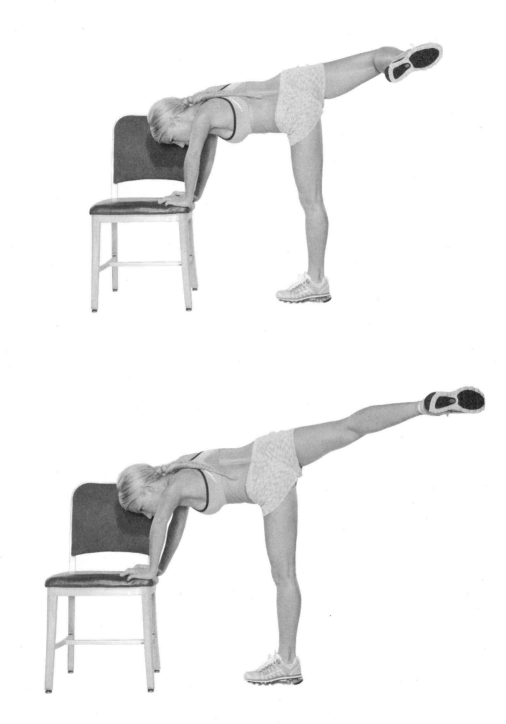

Move #42: Double Attitude Side Crunch

This is one of those moves where I'm going to be putting your body in a unique position to target a specific accessory muscle—in this case, it's in your abs. This one is tricky, because you're going to wrap your arm around your body.

Stance: Lie on the floor with your legs stretched out in front of you.

Action: Roll your body to the left, and place your right arm across your torso, fingertips on the floor. Extend your left arm straight out from your shoulder. Raise your left leg off the floor and bend your knee. Extend it straight out again, lift it to 180 degrees, and lower again. Toes are pointed the entire time.

Flow: In, extend low, high, lower. In, low, high, lower.

If you have to support your neck, you can take your left hand and put it behind your head.

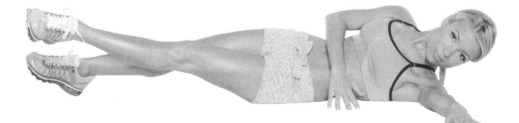

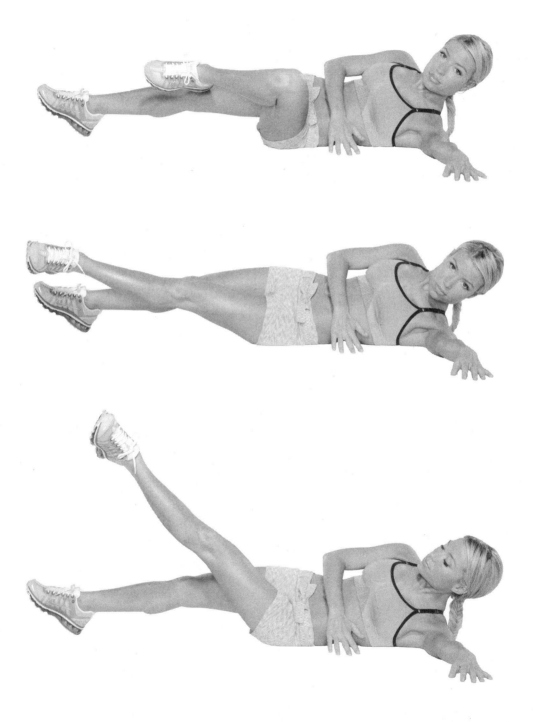

Move #43: Double Attitude Crunch with Arm Reach

A similar move to the one you just did, with an add-on for more challenge—and extra results.

Stance: Lie on the floor with your legs stretched out in front of you and lifted slightly off the ground. Extend your left hand way out from your shoulder, making a right angle with your arm and your torso, and reaching your fingers out on the floor, away from your body. Support your head with your right hand.

Action: Lift both legs up in attitude (knees bent to ninety degrees), crunching your left knee higher, toward your nose. Then straighten the legs, crossing your left ankle over your right ankle.

Flow: Lift and crunch, straighten and cross.

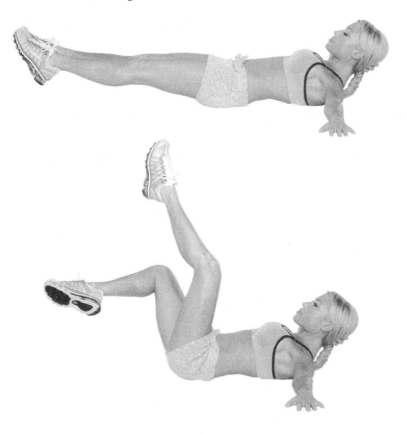

Move #44: Cross Right, Left, Right, Center Frog

You'll thank me for all this ab work later...

Stance: Lie on the floor with your legs stretched out in front of you, about shoulder width apart. Place your hands behind your head.

Action: Crunch up, supporting your head with your hands. Cross your straightened right leg over your left leg toward your left side, crossing the midline (if you drew a line from head to toe through your nose). Then cross your left leg over your right leg toward the right side, crossing the midline. Then cross the right leg over the left leg but stay in the center, and bend your legs up (like a frog) through the center, right ankle crossed over the left at the top, crunching as you frog. Straighten back to neutral (starting position).

Flow: Cross right to the right, left to the left, right in the center, crunch and frog. Right, left, right center, crunch and frog.

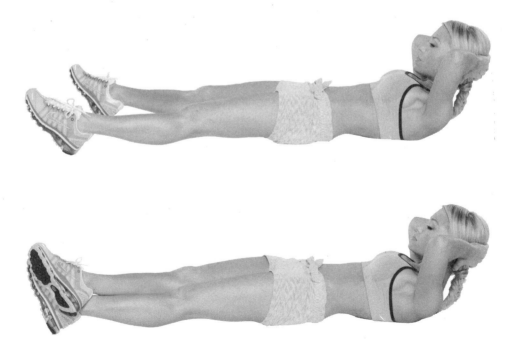

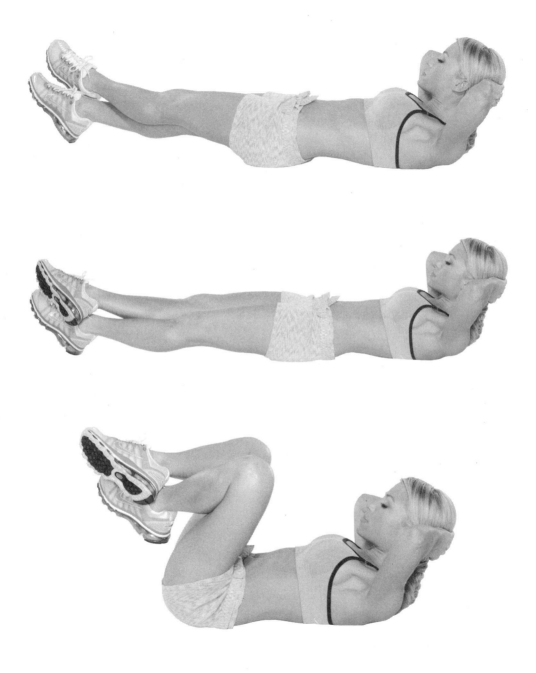

Move #45: Palms Forward Reach and Switch

For our final arm series, we're going to be standing.

Stance: Stand straight, arms out to the sides, fingers extended, palms open and forward. Bend your right arm in at the elbow.

Action: Reach out with your right arm, keeping the fingers wide and the palms open to the front of the room. Reach to the side, pull back in and bend, reach diagonally up, pull back in.

This move relies on rib isolations. Keep your hips still and where they are, and move your ribs over your hips in little isolated movements. That's going to work with your arms. When your arm reaches to the right, the hip goes to the left, but the rib goes to the right. The cross-vector of force is in the exchanging of the weight from the right to the left.

Flow: Reach to the side, back, reach diagonally up, back. Two times on the right and two times on the left.

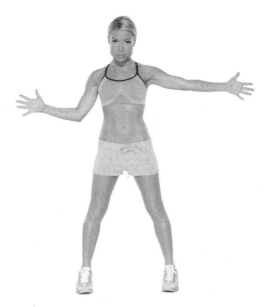

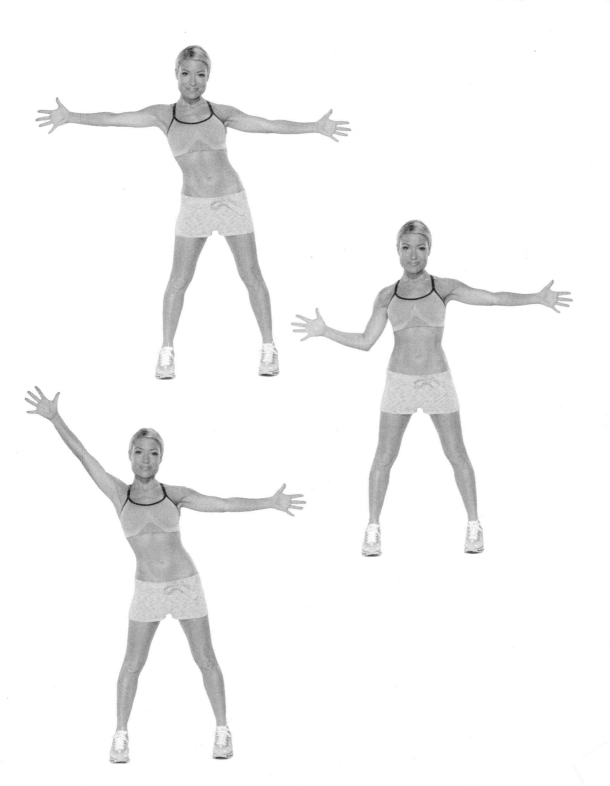

Move #46: Forward Press and Push

No more relaxing one of your arms while you're moving the other—in this move, both arms stay active. Keep your left arm extended while you work the right arm, and vice versa.

Stance: Stand straight with your arms reaching to the sides, fingers extended, palms open and forward. Feet can turn in slightly.

Action: With your left arm stretching actively to the side, reach your right arm out, palm facing forward. With your right arm, do a small press forward, and then a big reach forward.

Flow: Small press and reach. Press and reach.

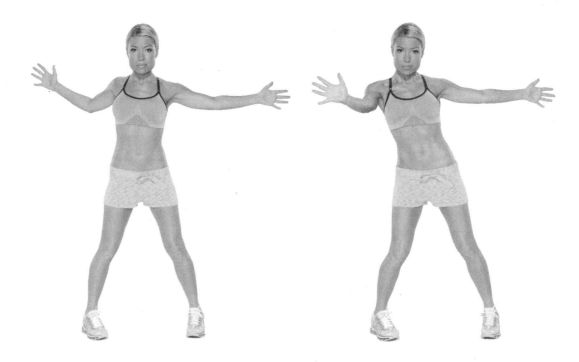

Move #47: Wide Reach Up, Back, and Forward

This move has a large range of motion, so get ready to work your shoulders. Remember to reach for the back when your arms are up and at your sides.

Stance: Stand tall, arms straight up from your shoulders and back, in a wide V. Your palms should be facing the sides of the room.

Action: Bring your arms down to shoulder height, turning your palms over as you do so they are facing up when your arms reach shoulder height. Thumbs should be moving toward the back of the room so you are really working your shoulders. Swing your arms forward so they are extended straight in front of you, palms facing up, thumbs pointing to the sides of the room. Then swing your arms back to shoulder height at your sides and back up to a wide V (as in Photo 1) with your palms facing down to the sides, pinkies reaching for the back of the room.

Flow: Up, sides, forward, sides. Up, sides, forward, sides.

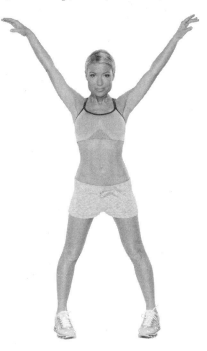

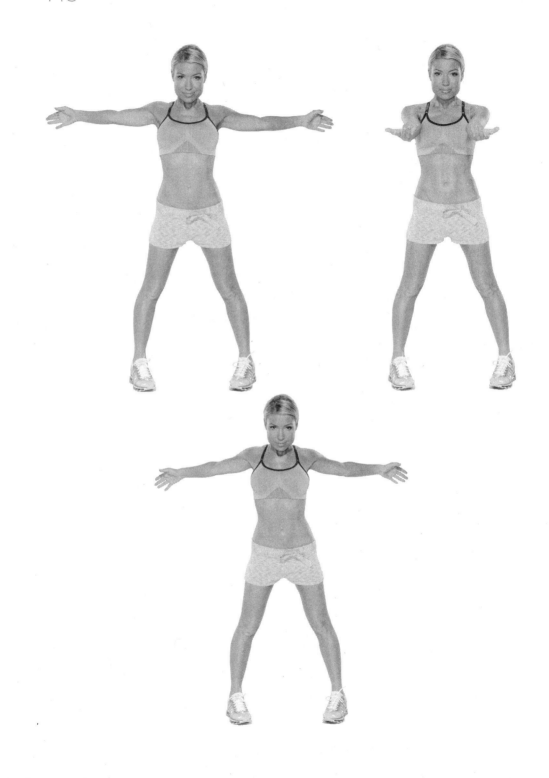

Move #48: Arms Forward Hit 1, 2, 3 with Arm Sweep Back

Don't just wiggle your hands at the wrist—really hit in this move. Hitting with force activates muscles that merely waving your hands misses.

Stance: Stand tall with both arms extended in front of you, palms facing to the right when you're working your right side. Toes turned in slightly. This is neutral.

Action: You are going to "hit" by sweeping your arms in a hitting motion. Hit in front of you at shoulder height, move back to neutral, then reach up above you and hit, and then hit at shoulder height again—1, 2, 3. Then turn your palm to the side, leading with the wrist, and sweep your arm straight all the way behind you.

Flow: Hit in front, above, in front, and then use your momentum to sweep your wrist back. And repeat.

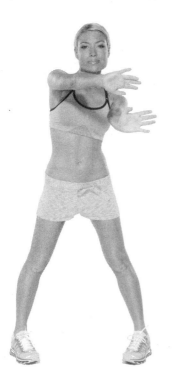
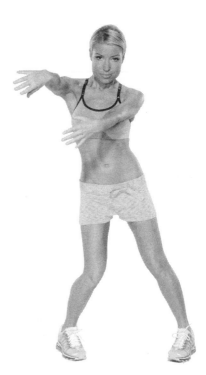

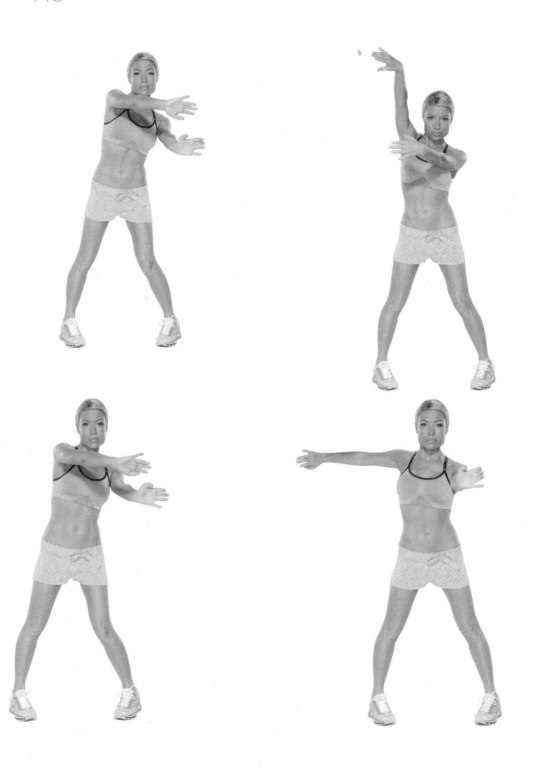

7

TA Method Cardio Complement

Performing the 30-Day Method Dance Aerobics

The second component of the 30-Day Method

is the Cardio Complement. In addition to the Muscle Design Work you'll be doing every day during your kick start, you'll also be doing daily cardio routines. The cardio portion of this 30-Day boot camp is integral for your weight loss. It is what will help your body burn off all the excess fat while you redesign your muscles on the mat and you learn to eat right by following my menus.

You might notice that this chapter is shorter than the others. That doesn't make it less important. Since dancing isn't something that can be communicated effectively with just words and still pictures, I decided it would be best to include a DVD with some follow-along steps that you can do at home. The DVD contains two routines, each ten minutes long, and it contains all the tools you need to work out at the appropriate intensity for your fitness level. More on that in a minute...

All Cardio Is Not Created Equal

Calories in, calories out. That's a fact. But the way we rid our bodies of stored energy is the key to reshaping our bodies to the desired physical outcome—in this case, a trim, slim, sexy, feminine figure.

While most workout programs advise doing cardio, often they are not particular about what kind. Running, Spin classes—these types of cardio might get your heart rate up, and they might burn calories, but they are not TA Method approved.

The typical cardiovascular exercises, like running, elliptical, biking, and so on, work the same muscles over and over again, bulking up certain muscle groups, ignoring others, and causing stress on your joints. When you do the same movement over and over, not only are you putting wear and tear on your joints, but you are also making your large muscles do exactly what they're trained to do. Grow bigger.

With my Cardio Complement, as you will see on the DVD, we practice a diverse range of movements. We don't rinse, repeat, rinse, repeat. The Method Cardio introduces you to choreography that combines jumping with movements that activate every muscle in your body. Everything has to help you twist, turn, reach, balance. Dancers, gymnasts, martial artists, the acrobats you marvel at when you go to the Cirque du Soleil—their strength doesn't come from repetition but from variation. By moving your body in all directions, I can still target your moves for efficiency and toning instead of building the horse muscle groups with the type of repetitive movements that happen when you run, climb stairs, or bike.

You've Got to Keep on Moving

A lean physique comes not just from activity but from *continuous* activity. I have been a dancer since I was three. What I have realized over the years is how ineffective stop-and-go training is when it comes to cardio.

When you are a dancer, classes move in an instructional stop-and-go curriculum. That is not effective for weight loss—and it's one of the reasons I was able to *gain* weight while I was at a school for dance. Whenever you have a performance run, everybody loses weight, because performances are not stop-and-go instruction but a continuous flow and release of energy. This knowledge has always informed my dance aerobics.

I started my dance aerobics more than a decade ago, and throughout the development of my Method, its principles remain constant. My training as a dancer makes me appreciate not only how movement represents itself within the body—by burning energy through continuous movement, and by knitting the muscles together through varied movement—but also how the movements translate aesthetically. My cardio is not just jumping around—it is actually dancing, the kind of movements that can be choreographed into the longer routines you will find on my more advanced DVDs.

I love dancing. And eventually, when your endurance increases, you will find yourself loving it, too. The body wants to move, and once you release it there will be no holding you back.

You Must Commit to the Cardio Complement!

With this DVD, you'll learn to leap, to turn, to kick, going in one direction and then changing it up. Since this is a 30-Day boot camp, instead of providing complex choreography for you to learn, which would result in stop-and-go exercise, I've given you two series of combined movements that you can perform continuously while your endurance increases and you shed the weight. While you do the moves, you are also revisiting the specific angles that promote the musculostructure design changes you're making, making sure that while you are burning calories at a very high rate, you are always toning instead of bulking.

During this 30-Day challenge, I am asking you to surrender your body to me. No more Spinning class. No more running. I am not saying you can never participate in these activities again. I am simply stating that doing these activities during your focused daily workout time is not going to give you the results you want.

In order to reach your goals, you need to do cardio regularly—but it has to be *my* cardio. If you opt out of the dance cardio and try to replace it with something else, you will not be following my program, and your results will be affected. But if you stick with my Cardio Complement, and you do the Muscle Design, and you follow the menus, your results will amaze you.

The Benefits of the Method Cardio

My dance aerobics is a cardiovascular energizing activity that has many important benefits. It will help you burn the maximum amount of fat and calories and positively affect your skin tone, your endurance, your overall health, your emotional health—and even your sex life!

Maximum Fat and Calorie Burning: The Method Cardio is designed so your body can burn the maximum fat and calories possible during the time allotted. With my cardio, your entire body is engaged, not just the lower half, as on many machines. Even your brain gets involved, because you're using different movements, not just a repetitive running or cycling motion. And unlike other kinds of exercise—tennis, golf, or your typical stop-and-start aerobics classes—it relies on continuous motion, so you get real results, fast.

Skin Tone: My cardio is essential for getting the skin back to the muscle after you've redesigned your structure to a streamlined frame. When I say "getting the skin back to the muscle," I'm talking about eradicating the bane of women everywhere: the dreaded cellulite. Want to banish cottage cheese thighs from your life forever? Do your cardio every day.

Endurance: By using my Cardio Complement, you are also increasing your endurance while you encourage all the positive changes you started with your Muscle Design, working your muscles strategically to tighten and tone instead of just making your muscles bigger. It is endurance that will allow you to really do all the prescribed moves and routines correctly. Once you can successfully perform twenty minutes of cardio, you won't dread your workouts anymore. And once you can successfully perform forty minutes of my dance cardio, you will be well on your way to a real lifestyle change.

Physical Health: Every time you do my cardio, you sweat and detoxify. Your skin will have a new glow, and you will have a new spring in your step. Meanwhile, you are improving your heart and lung capacity. You are reducing your chances of getting illnesses such as heart disease and cancer. And, especially important for women, you are taking care of your bones and preventing diseases like osteoporosis. How's that for a side effect?

Emotional Health: Feeling amazing isn't just about looking good—it's about feeling good. By developing your endurance and strengthening your muscles, you will change the way you feel in your own skin. You will be in a better mood. You will feel more confident. You will even sleep better!

Your Sex Life! By mastering the dance routines, by learning to control the way your muscles move and work together, you will have a new awareness of the way your body moves, and this awareness will translate into transformation in so many areas of your life…Not only will you own your new figure, but you will be more graceful and your movements will be more purposeful and elegant. Many of my clients tell me that their sex lives get a boost because they feel sexier!

Be Religious

What I hear from many of my clients is that at the outset, cardio is not usually anyone's favorite. There are exceptions, but by and large learning to perform the cardio well is a struggle for everyone. It doesn't happen overnight. Doing it every day helps, however. And the better you get, the happier you will be to do it. I promise you that once you're used to the physical exertion, you can relax and just really enjoy yourself. One of my clients, who used to complain every time she walked into my studio that she wasn't "in the mood," confessed to me recently that after her endurance improved, she started thinking about cardio as "going dancing" instead of "exercising."

Depending on your level of physical fitness, it can take a few days or a few weeks to get really comfortable with the cardio. Because let's be honest: It isn't like going to a spa. It isn't like sitting back and relaxing while somebody fixes you a cup of tea. It is work—hard, physical work that can be uncomfortable at the get-go.

If you skip days in between your cardio workouts, your body forgets how good it can feel to really sweat. It works against you instead of with you, telling you that missing just a day, just two days, won't make a difference in the long run. Don't tell yourself that you can make up for missed time. You can't. Time is worth more than money—the time you spend working out is an investment in yourself, in your health, and in the way you will feel when you wake up every day from now on.

What I have found is that if you don't make your cardio a consistent daily practice, you are likely to make up an excuse within the first five minutes of starting. Sure, you have good intentions—so you schedule your workout. You get dressed and prepare your environment. You start moving. It's uncomfortable. Your mind starts to list all the reasons why right now isn't really convenient. You try to talk yourself into staying motivated, because after all, you want to look better and be healthier.

Ten minutes later, you've turned off your playlist and you're back to checking e-mail.

The above scenario is not the way to get the job done. Cardio is like doing the dishes. If you deal with them right away, then the task is easy; if you let them pile up, it's a lot more work and a lot more annoying. It's much easier to do a little bit of cardio every day than step on the scale and realize that ten pounds have turned into twenty.

If you work out every day, you will learn to expect the little voice that tells you *Stop*, and you will learn to talk over it. Your body will get used to sweating, and it will crave it. Besides, training consistently isn't just better for your results. It's also healthier for your joints. Once you incorporate the Cardio Complement into your regular schedule, your body will be fluid and ready for movement, which will help prevent injuries, so you can keep moving toward your goals, literally!

How to Maximize Your Cardio Time

We've already talked about how to set up your space for optimal working out. For the cardio, as you'll remember, you want a room with hardwood floors, if possible. And remember to keep the room warm. No AC! You're here to sweat! Lace up your ship-shape sneakers, line up your mirrors, get the couch out of the way—and get moving. The key is constant movement. This is not a stop–start activity—it is meant to be a continuous cycle of pure energy burning.

The DVD demonstrates the moves you will use during your cardio workout. I want you to learn the moves, and then I want you to really dance. To burn the most calories and fat during your allotted cardio time, you have to be a true cardiovascular performer. That means you can't mess around. No mindless, halfway jumping, no checking your watch or dreaming about lunch.

Think about when you watch your favorite performers. You want to watch, because they're engaging everything they have. They own what they are doing, and they show it to the world. If you want to see results, you have to bring that same professional mentality to your cardio routine. Treat every session as if you're auditioning for the biggest role of your life. Or playing the championship game. Because you know what? You are. This is your time to lose weight—your time to be the best you. And I promise, the rewards are well worth it!

How to Get to Peak Level No Matter Where You're at Now

First things first: Always consult your health care professional before beginning any cardio program. But even if you aren't already addicted to cardio, this book is for you. No matter what your current fitness level is, you can use this program to get yourself into better shape. The cardio DVD that I have included is 100 percent doable. You will not need to learn routines or memorize choreography. The moves are designed so you can launch in with no experience and still get all the benefits. You will increase your endurance, burn calories and fat, and set yourself up for continued future success.

What If I'm Not a Great Dancer? Will I Be Able to Do This?

You do not need to be a great dancer, a good dancer, or even a dancer at all to master this cardio. We all have natural rhythms in us. If you can walk, you can do this. Just remember that learning to do dance aerobics if you've never tried it can feel like learning a new language. Gwyneth Paltrow, Courtney Cox, and Molly Sims all looked puzzled at the thought of having to learn dance aerobics in the beginning. None of them was a dancer, and now they are all amazing at it! They, like you, had to invest the time and energy. If dance aerobics is a language, they have learned to speak it fluently. And so can you!

Ultimately, I want you to repeat the entire DVD (both combinations) two times with jumping, which equals forty minutes of cardio. If you aren't used to prolonged cardio, this is going to be an adventure for you—one that is going to really pay off in the end.

Getting Started

If you are not used to jumping in your exercise routines, then I ask that you begin by following the first combination on the DVD without jumping. Simply step-touch the moves as described below, pushing yourself toward increased endurance.

You'll use the lower-impact step-touching technique until you can repeat the whole DVD twice for the full forty minutes, and then move on to jumping, replacing step-touching with jumping in ten-minute increments every three days. Below, you'll find Start Charts for four different fitness levels: absolute beginners, moderate beginners, intermediate, and advanced.

Once the forty minutes is easy for you, you can make a sixty-minute playlist and repeat the combinations as needed—but you really shouldn't go over an hour of cardio a day. It's not sustainable, and it's not necessary. If you recalibrate your body to need more than that, you're setting yourself up for time management issues.

ABSOLUTE BEGINNER START CHART

Days 1–3	If you never exercise at all, you'll begin by step-touching Combination 1 on the DVD. If you are really out of shape, remember, no jumping!
Days 4–6	Step-touch the entire DVD, no jumping, for a total of 20 minutes of step-touching.
Days 7–9	Step-touch the entire DVD and then repeat Combination 1, for a total of 30 minutes of step-touching.
Days 10–12	Step-touch the entire DVD twice. Total time: 40 minutes.

Days 13–15   Incorporate jumping into your routine: Jump through Combination 1, and then step-touch for the additional 30 minutes.

Days 16–18   Jump through the DVD, and then step-touch for the additional 20 minutes.

Days 19–21   30 minutes of jumping, 10 minutes of step-touching.

Days 22–30   You have pushed yourself to full-octane cardio! 40 minutes of jumping. If the 40 minutes becomes easy for you, create a 60-minute playlist—but don't go over 60 minutes per day.

MODERATE BEGINNER START CHART

Days 1–3   Those who "walk but don't run" will step-touch the entire DVD twice for the first 3 days.

Days 4–6   Incorporate jumping into your routine: Jump through Combination 1, and then step-touch for the additional 30 minutes.

Days 7–9   Jump through the DVD, and then step-touch for the additional 20 minutes.

Days 10–12   30 minutes of jumping, 10 minutes of step-touching.

Days 13–15   Congratulations! You have pushed yourself to 40 minutes of jumping. If the 40 minutes becomes easy for you, create a 60-minute playlist—but don't go over 60 minutes per day.

INTERMEDIATE START CHART

Days 1–3   Moderate athletes begin by jumping through the routines as shown on the DVD. Jump for 20 minutes, and then step-touch for 20 minutes.

Days 4–6   30 minutes of jumping, 10 minutes of step-touching.

Days 7–9   You have achieved full-octane cardio! 40 minutes of jumping. If the 40 minutes becomes easy for you, create a 60-minute playlist— but don't go over 60 minutes per day.

ADVANCED START CHART

Days 1–3   If you're already very athletic, begin by jumping through the routines as shown on the DVD. Jump through the entire DVD twice. Remember to really perform!

Days 4–30   If the 40 minutes becomes easy for you, create a 60-minute playlist—but don't go over 60 minutes per day.

How to Avoid and Deal with Common Injuries

If you've ever seen athletes hobbling around on crutches, or the office marathoner sporting an Ace bandage, you already know that physical activities can be harmful to our bodies if we aren't careful. (This is one reason I advise getting a new pair of sneakers that will give you proper cushioning and support.)

The three main symptoms that may crop up while you're getting used to the cardio are shin splints, side cramps, and, at the beginning, exhaustion.

Shin Splints are a nasty, but common, complaint of runners and dancers. Prolonged jumping can injure the muscles or eventually induce tiny stress fractures in the shinbones. To prevent shin splints, make sure your sneakers are offering you the proper support, and make sure you are doing your daily stretches. If you get shin splints, back off from jumping but not from doing your cardio entirely. If you feel symptoms, which include tenderness along the shins on either the inside or the outside of the leg, warm the room up more and do the DVD without jumping. Two days without jumping should do it. As soon as you're feeling better, try jumping again.

Side Cramps are a sign that you are pushing yourself and, therefore, building up your endurance. Don't work through a side cramp. Listen to your body telling you that you need to take a break for a moment. Stop and walk around the room, then start back up when it goes away, but make sure not to use it as an excuse to quit. If side cramps are a persistent issue, you might try adding some potassium to your diet. (When I need more potassium, I mix half a Zico coconut water with regular H_2O and enjoy as a potassium-enriched workout drink.)

Exhaustion is something you can expect to feel at the beginning of your cardio program. For the first few days, you will feel like a ton of bricks. You may crave a nap, or find yourself going to bed at 9 p.m. But later, you will feel lighter on your feet. Your workouts will leave you feeling energized instead of wiped out. And eventually, the energy will last all day long...

Get Inspired by the Music!

The music you listen to while you work out is extremely important. Each combination is set to music, but feel free to put it on mute and use your own playlist. (I've listed some of my favorite tunes at the end of this chapter.) Eventually, you want your playlist to be forty minutes long. You want it to be fast-paced; you want it to get your feet moving. In my studio, I make sure that we always have up-to-date iPods to keep us inspired. The music you choose for your cardio is going to reflect how excited you are to show up each day. Most people don't think they're going to love to do their cardio. But a great playlist helps. And once you get good at it, trust me, it's going to be one of your favorite things to do.

Tracy's Cardio Playlist

"In the Sun" (JAW Breakers Remix), Michael Stipe with Chris Martin

"Diva" (Karmatronic Club Remix), Beyoncé

"Circus" (Villains Remix), Britney Spears

"Don't Stop the Music" (The Wideboys Club Mix), Rihanna

"Read My Mind" (Pet Shop Boys "Stars Are Blazing" Mix), the Killers

"Sober" (Bimbo Jones Extended Club Mix), Pink

"Boom Boom Boom" (DJ Ammo/Poet Named Life Megamix), Black Eyed Peas

"Love Sex Magic" (Jason Nevins Sex Club Mix), Ciara featuring Justin Timberlake

"Talk" (Thin White Duke Mix), Coldplay

Work It

When you're doing your cardio, don't be afraid to really push yourself. Don't stop the second you feel uncomfortable. Wait for that second wave of energy to carry you through. You need to sweat every day, and this is your time to make that happen.

8

TA Method Menus

Healthy, Delicious Meals to Power Your Weight Loss

The third and final part of the 30-Day Method is my meal plan. As I mentioned earlier, this specifically designed eating blueprint is absolutely essential to the 30-Day Method. Exercise alone is not going to get rid of the extra weight that you came to this book with. The good news is that these menus will help you shed the pounds, creating a clean slate so that I can redesign your body, improve your health, and give you the tools for long-term sustainability.

The menus work in conjunction with the cardio and muscle work, so unlike the here-today, gone-tomorrow effects of fad diets you may have tried in the past, you will own your new body. And it won't be skinny fat, the way just dieting works. It will be fit, toned, tight, healthy—and all yours. By following my menu plan, you will be supporting all your intensive cardio work for maximum fat burning while the Muscle Design reshapes your structure. In addition, my plan will teach you how to make positive eating choices well beyond thirty days.

Food is everywhere. And it isn't just about nutrition for most of us—eating is social and emotional as well as physical. Have you ever noticed that many people who don't feel great about their bodies also do not have positive associations with eating? And often, people who are happy with their bodies have very positive associations with food.

That's because when we eat clean, nutritious foods, we actually restore the chemical balance that we're supposed to have in our bodies. We then feel better and begin to naturally gravitate to the foods we are naturally supposed to be eating.

Relearning How to Eat

A balanced eating plan is imperative for healthy weight loss. When you change your eating habits permanently, when you commit to a healthier lifestyle, you eliminate the chaos that yo-yo dieting can bring into your life. I wanted to create a weight loss nutritional program that satisfies cravings, gives you mental clarity, and offers a path to physical transformation.

The menus I've developed with the help of John Byrne, executive chef for the Tracy Anderson Method, will play a large part in improving your skin tone, physique, and overall health. Being on a "diet" can have so many negative connotations…instead, consider these menus part of your self-renewal and conscious lifestyle change. They will help you kick-start your weight loss and get you on the right track. Ultimately, I want you to rediscover your relationship with food so that you can sit at the table and relax and socialize without worrying about how it will impact your weight. But for the first thirty days, you are going to need to follow these menus to a T if you want to see real results.

In this book, I offer two menu plans to help you jump-start your weight loss and results. For the first twenty-five days of your kick start, you will enjoy the Lifestyle Menus: delicious, easy-to-prepare foods that will work perfectly with even the busiest of schedules. For the final five days, you will power up to a strong finish with my Cleanse Menu, designed to help you shed the weight while you still enjoy real foods with no mixes or powders.

Since the body is a reflection of what we eat and how we move, the foods we eat and the exercises we choose have a direct relationship with our energy levels and the shape of our bodies. It's as simple as that. If we make every dietary choice a calculated one and every workout a Workout with a capital *W*, then the results will be visible for all to see.

That's why it's essential for you to stick with me and truly commit to changing your lifestyle and detoxing from your bad habits, and to adopting a fresh new way of moving, living—and eating, which I'm about to describe. Trust me—after three weeks on these menus, if you eat processed foods, you're going to feel it, and it very likely won't feel good to you. Once your body gets used to regular infusions of fresh, unprocessed, highly nutritious foods, you won't want to go back to your old styles of eating.

Healthy Eating Means Balance

Earlier in the book, I described my obsessive quest to find the most effective way to exercise in order to change the body's shape. Well, about a decade ago, I also started researching the impact that nutrition can have on the body. I was responsible for navigating 150 women with different habits, styles, and needs along the path to perfection, so I had to understand how food impacted the body and the weight loss process. And I started investigating the effects of nutrition beyond weight loss, for the purpose of health, vitality, and longevity.

I tried a raw food diet, where I ate completely raw for four months. It didn't work for me. My skin was good. But I stopped menstruating, and I became very, very thin. I've been a vegetarian. I've been vegan. I've tried eating comfort food, eating in moderation, and I've overindulged. I've tried it all, really. And I learned what works and what doesn't.

Listen, I am definitely not someone who likes to diet. My engagement with food is a true affair of the heart. I grew up in the Midwest, eating meat and potatoes. My mom *never* allowed us to eat junk food—which of course just increased my desire for it. I would go over to my friend's house and dive for the "Ding Dong" drawer. That's how I learned that, even with junk food, we want to find a balance, and avoid words like *never*.

I like cheeseburgers, and crave a steak and mashed potatoes and creamed spinach sometimes. I'm not one of those people who say, "I don't understand why people need cake every night." Or, "I don't understand how someone could eat twenty Double Stuff Oreos."

Food is a big part of living and enjoying. Paula Deen is one of my heroes. I do not promote diet-for-life or fad diets. When you travel, you want to be able to sample the delicious food available. When you're home, you want to be able to gather at a table with your family, not obsess over calories. So by no means do I ever want to promote a nutrition solution for the perfect you that is based on never enjoying the many joys that come with eating.

The key is balance.

The Basis for the Method Menus

I developed these menus in the custom style that I approach my fitness method. I've been there, so I understand where you are weak. I understand where you're coming from. And I have menus to help you. I'm not promoting a raw-is-the-only-way, vegetarian-is-the-only-way, meat-eating-is-the-only-way, cutting-carbs-is-the-only-way kind of approach. I'm not promoting any one thing. Instead, I've cherry-picked the best elements of the best approaches to eating to pull together a truly unique and satisfying way of feeding ourselves.

In designing the menus, I had a few important bottom-line goals: using *real food*, with all the benefits that come from eating whole and not processed foods; paying attention to *digestion*, for the full absorption of nutrients and phytochemicals; and choosing a menu plan that would deliver maximum *satisfaction*.

Real Food

The recipes in these menus all use fresh fruits and vegetables: apples, kale, kiwis, chestnuts, carrots, to name a few. Even when it's time for your five-day cleanse, you'll still be enjoying delicious menu options that are not mixed from powders or supplements. These days, the big processed food companies are jumping on the "superfood" trend but not delivering "superfood" nutrients. We have been programmed to trust brands that appear to represent health, but we have to retrain ourselves and realize that *real food* can be convenient and healthy. The foods on this menu start at the farm and make it to your table with no stops in a factory to be dosed with preservatives or other unhealthy additives, or sealed in cellophane. We do not use food substitutes or flavor substitutes: There is, after all, no substitute for real flavor.

The National Cancer Institute begs us to consume more fruits and vegetables, which contain phytochemicals, the keys to preventing some of our most life-threatening diseases, not to mention the benefits they provide for our beauty and longevity. Juicing has become popular because it helps us digest enough phytochemicals to reap real benefits. The menus provide recipes for green juices that will give you energy and all the phytochemicals you need to reap the benefits of these powerhouse nutrients, which can only be found in real food.

Digestion

When thinking about nutrition for the 30-Day Kick Start, I took a look at the commonsense way we feed young children. We don't stuff them full of goodies one day and then starve them the next—we would consider that to be abuse. Instead, we make sure to feed them every few hours on a regular schedule so they are never fussy. They digest their food slowly but are never overloaded. With the Kick-Start Menus, you'll be eating digestible combinations of delicious, healthful foods that will keep your blood sugar levels even so you don't crash and burn in the middle of the afternoon.

The menus are designed to undo the damage you have done to your body, eliminate any extra weight you have when you begin my Method, and give you maximum energy so that you can really perform your Cardio Complement and Muscle Design Work.

Satisfaction

I also thought about how and why we eat (and overeat). I dedicated a *year* to perfecting chocolate desserts made of real food that have no weight gain culprit in them. Because I understand how detrimental fake desserts are. And how important it is to feel satisfied by delicious foods.

Many people tend to overeat for any number of reasons—boredom, stress, extra-lengthy holiday meals. Now you're going to learn how to eat to power your body. As you use the menus, keep in mind: The suggested portion sizes will provide the fastest results. But if you're still hungry, I encourage you to eat a larger portion. I do not want you to be walking around hungry. I need you to have enough energy to really perform.

If you aren't used to eating healthfully, you may find that you feel hungry while your body acclimates to eating fresh, natural foods. I do not control your portions, so you may always have some more of the prescribed foods if you need it. But keep in mind that in order to gain the weight, you spent some time feeling uncomfortably overstuffed. Overeating and convenience foods tend not to satisfy but to stupefy. So if you feel hungry on this eating plan, make sure you really need nutrition and not just the familiar comfort of another bite. The menus are calibrated to give you enough nutrition and calories, so just have a hot tea and learn a new way of comfort that doesn't have to do with food—and the satisfaction that comes with eating right and looking and feeling great.

How to Use the TA Method Menus

The TA Method Menu Plan has two phases and is intended for thirty days. During your kick start, you must make every effort to not stray from the foods listed in the menus. Over the course of this program, the muscular work is changing your structure, and the cardio is burning fat and getting the skin back to the muscle. The menus are here to support all the good work you're doing—so no substitutions, unless absolutely necessary.

You'll see that our menus call for kefir yogurt in place of regular yogurt. While all yogurt with live cultures is good for you, kefir yogurt has even more healthy bacteria to keep your digestive tract healthy. The same goes for yacón syrup, which can be purchased at higher-end markets. Yacón syrup is delicious, sweet—and has only half the calories of maple syrup.

While you're preparing your meals, make sure not to add any additional fats or oils during the cooking process. We use an organic olive oil spray that is a zero-fat product. When sautéing or grilling, just spray that onto the pan, not onto the food.

We only have thirty days, so let's make them count!

Days 1–25: Tracy's Lifestyle and Vegetarian Lifestyle Menus

For the first twenty-five days of your kick start, you will enjoy one of these menus, both collections of my lifestyle favorites, with flavorful recipes for soups, salads, entrées, and, yes, chocolatey desserts. You can expect to lose three to five pounds per week on the Lifestyle Menus. These menus avoid the common diet-spoiling culprits, like sugar and processed foods, that cause people to gain weight, have mood swings, and experience health problems.

The Lifestyle Menus offer sensible, healthy portions that remove the confusion for those times when you need a little bit of extra help. Protein doesn't come from powder but from delicious, nutritious Chicken Protein or Tofu Vegetable Soup. As you learn to perform cardiovascularly, these specially designed menus will support your transformation.

Days 26–30: Tracy's Performance Cleanse Menu

For the final five days of your kick start, you're going to shift to my Performance Cleanse to detox your system and show off newly sculpted muscles. The Cleanse offers filling food that powers your body with impactful nutrients that promote fat loss, make your skin glow, and give you energy. With the Cleanse, you can expect to lose five to nine pounds in a week. The Cleanse Menu is not a liquid diet, but offers fresh fruit and vegetable smoothie-style puddings and meal choices to give you energy while you detox and shed the weight.

I put the Cleanse at the end because I want you to be really successful. Shifting from your regular styles of eating to an intense detox—at the same time that you are beginning a new exercise program—takes more willpower than most people have, and really just sets you up for failure. By incorporating healthier eating for twenty-five days before your detox, you are nurturing yourself toward sustainable weight loss and improved health.

Days 31 and Beyond

After the thirty days, you can turn to the menus as needed to keep you in your amazing new weight zone. As you integrate fully into my system, as long as you are consistently doing the workouts, your body will be recalibrated to exist in a totally different state. Eventually, your new way of eating will become a healthy, unconscious habit instead of a series of conscious choices. When it comes to food, for regular maintenance, I use the 80/20 rule: 80 percent commitment to targeted nutrition, 20 percent guilt-free enjoyment.

Who can love life if you're always counting food points?

Make a Change Instead of an Excuse!

Taking care of our inner and outer beauty requires our focus and attention. And it can be time consuming, especially when we're working to change the effects of decades of unconscious behavior. A busy schedule is one of the most common excuses that people make for not taking proper care of themselves.

Look around you. Who do you know that isn't too busy, jam-packed, over-scheduled? The food industry knows how harried you feel, and how that translates to mealtimes. But the quick and easy, ultra-convenient food choices, like fast food and overly processed packaged foods, while they may seem like a perfect solution for overburdened schedules, are the opposite. They don't help you—they hurt you. Extra weight, that feeling of bloat that won't seem to go away, nutrient deficiency, higher blood pressure, heart disease—these are some of the near and far "benefits" of convenience foods.

If it's your workload that is your "I'm too busy" excuse, keep in mind that eating poorly reflects clearly in the way you look and feel—and so does eating well. If you follow my guidelines, you will soon see how treating your system to the highest-quality nutrition gives you the energy to consistently do your best. Do you truly want to be successful? Then make time for proper nutrition and consistent exercise.

If your kids are your go-to "I would if I could" story, well, how about setting a good example when you set the table? Obesity is at a global high. Childhood obesity is on the rise. And there's no better way to teach your children about eating healthfully and exercising regularly than setting a good example. So let's get to it!

Tracy's Lifestyle Menu and Vegetarian Lifestyle Menu: Days 1–25

During the first twenty-five days of your kick start, you're going to follow the Lifestyle Menu or the Vegetarian Lifestyle Menu, both of which are highly nutritious and satisfying weight loss food plans. In order to get you started on your path to eating right, every day, I've made the menus as simple as possible to make sure you can follow them easily and get the best results. Everything is clearly laid out so that you can learn how to prepare flavorful, satisfying foods while avoiding the junk that we usually add—like sugar, salt, and oils—without even thinking about it.

In my experience, when people start a new diet, having too many choices leads to confusion. I don't want you to spend your time wondering what to eat, when, or why. It is for this reason that I do not offer a row of daily choices. This menu is a twenty-five-day prescription, so I need you to eat what I prescribe. Right now, instead of having your brain searching for what it wants to eat, I am reprogramming your brain to crave differently. Later, when you learn to want the right foods, you will be able to enjoy making choices. But when it comes to your kick start, you don't need to think about it—you just need to follow the instructions. We've carefully calibrated the menus so that you get the proper balance of nutrition every single day. No skipping or substituting!

While your body is processing all the work you've been doing, you're going to support that work by eating foods that will give you fuel and maintain your energy level while helping you lose weight. Along the way, you will learn to monitor your intake and pay attention to portion size, while making sure to eat enough so that you aren't hungry.

Remember, as we talked about, what "hungry" means to you is going to evolve throughout this program. On your way to gaining the extra weight, you were learning to overeat and confuse "overstuffed" with "satiated." Now you're learning to eat the right amount, which means never, ever feeling too full. I do not want you to be starving and irritable, low-energy, unable to summon the willpower to put on your sneakers. I want you to eat enough to be energized, vital, and ready to really perform.

As always, you'll want to consult with your doctor before starting any new eating plan. And if you're a vegetarian, make sure to take your usual supplements to get all the important nutrients you need, like B vitamins and iron.

REGULAR 25-DAY MEAL PLAN

DAY 1	DAY 2	DAY 3	DAY 4	DAY 5
Breakfast Strawberry Mint Salad (p. 240)	**Breakfast** Turkey Avocado Roll-Up (p. 222) with Wilted Spinach (p. 235)	**Breakfast** Veggie Omelet Roll-Up (p. 208)	**Breakfast** Berry Compote (p. 236)	**Breakfast** Halved Grapefruit (p. 238)
Lunch Tomato Minestrone Soup (p. 192)	**Lunch** Spinach Salad with Chestnuts (p. 203)	**Lunch** Grilled Salmon Salad with Endive and Red Onion (p. 201)	**Lunch** Chicken Protein Soup (p. 190)	**Lunch** Grilled Chicken with Broccoli and Endive (p. 211)
Snack Choco Chestnut Pudding (p. 241)	**Snack** Cucumber Mint Relish (p. 229)	**Snack** Blueberry Apple-sauce (p. 236)	**Snack** Kiwi Dessert (p. 242)	**Snack** Beet Salad with Oranges (p. 197)
Dinner Poached Cod (p. 216) and Roasted Aspara-gus (p. 232)	**Dinner** Steamed Turkey Breast with Wilted Kale and Raisins (p. 220)	**Dinner** Orange Glazed Salmon (p. 215) and Roasted Mush-rooms (p. 232)	**Dinner** Grilled Chicken with Mango and Scallion (p. 212)	**Dinner** Shrimp Salad with Sugar Snap Peas (p. 203)

DAY 6

Breakfast
Kale Juice
(p. 243) and a
hard-boiled egg

Lunch
Steamed Veggie
Plate (p. 234)

Snack
Honeydew Grape
Salad (p. 238)

Dinner
Seared Peppered
Tuna with Arugula
Greens (p. 219)

DAY 7

Breakfast
Mushroom
Omelet Roll-Up
(p. 206)

Lunch
Baked Chicken
with Broccoli
(p. 209)

Snack
Cucumber Mint
Relish (p. 229)

Dinner
Grilled Salmon
Salad with
Endive and Red
Onion (p. 201)
and Roasted
Triple Carrots
(p. 233)

DAY 8

Breakfast
Our "Bloody
Mary" (p. 244)

Lunch
Turkey Avocado
Roll-Up (p. 222)

Snack
Fresh Melon
Compote
(p. 237)

Dinner
Stovetop Braised
Red Snapper
(p. 220) and
Roasted
Asparagus
(p. 232)

DAY 9

Breakfast
Blueberries and
Blackberries
(p. 236)

Lunch
Puree of Broccoli
Soup (p. 190)

Snack
Beet Salad with
Oranges (p. 197)

Dinner
Roasted Turkey
and Steamed
Broccoli (p. 218)

DAY 10

Breakfast
Citrus Salad
(p. 237)

Lunch
Balsamic Chicken
Salad (p. 196)

Snack
Crudités with Dip
(p. 229)

Dinner
Poached Cod
(p. 216) and
Braised Leek
(p. 227)

DAY 11

Breakfast
Poached
Salmon Omelet
(p. 207)

Lunch
Grilled Chicken
over Fresh Spin-
ach Salad
(p. 200)

Snack
Choco Blueberry
Pudding (p. 241)

Dinner
Poached Cod
(p. 216) and
Roasted
Asparagus
(p. 232)

DAY 12

Breakfast
Citrus Salad
(p. 237)

Lunch
Roasted Root
Vegetables
(p. 232)

Snack
Cucumber Mint
Relish (p. 229)

Dinner
Turkey Burger
(p. 222) with
lettuce and
tomato

DAY 13

Breakfast
Veggie Omelet
Roll-Up (p. 208)

Lunch
Carrot Ginger
Soup (p. 189)

Snack
Blueberry Apple-
sauce (p. 236)

Dinner
Fillet of White
Fish with Olives
and Thyme
(p. 210)

DAY 14

Breakfast
Berry Compote
(p. 236)

Lunch
Seared Tilapia
with Lemon and
Mustard (p. 219)

Snack
Kiwi Dessert
(p. 242)

Dinner
Grilled Flank
Steak (p. 212)
and String Beans
with Sautéed
Spinach (p. 234)

DAY 15

Breakfast
Strawberry Mint
Salad (p. 240)

Lunch
Grilled Tofu over
White Romaine
Hearts (p. 201)

Snack
Beet Salad with
Oranges (p. 197)

Dinner
Orange Glazed
Salmon (p. 215)
with Corn and
Sweet Peppers
(p. 228)

DAY 16

Breakfast
Kefir Yogurt
(p. 242)

Lunch
Baked Sweet
Potato (p. 226)

Snack
Choco Chestnut
Pudding (p. 241)

Dinner
Grilled Lamb
Tenderloin
(p. 213) and
Roasted Brussels
Sprouts (p. 232)

DAY 17

Breakfast
Sweet Potato Sil-
ver Dollars Pan-
cakes with yacón
syrup (p. 221)

Lunch
Greek Salad with
Endive and Red
Onion (p. 198)

Snack
Pear Apple Spice
(p. 239)

Dinner
Steamed Turkey
Breast with
Wilted Kale and
Raisins (p. 220)

DAY 18

Breakfast
Tropical Fruit
Salad (p. 240)

Lunch
Turkey Kale Soup
(p. 193)

Snack
Choco Blueberry
Pudding (p. 241)

Dinner
Orange Glazed
Salmon (p. 215)
and Roasted
Mushrooms
(p. 232)

DAY 19

Breakfast
Mango Smoothie
(p. 242)

Lunch
Tuna Fish with
Roasted Cauli-
flower and Fennel
(p. 221)

Snack
Beet Salad with
Oranges (p. 197)

Dinner
Shrimp Salad
with Sugar Snap
Peas (p. 203)

DAY 20

Breakfast
Egg Spinach
Wrap (p. 205)

Lunch
Tofu Vegetable
Soup with Kale
and Swiss Chard
(p. 191)

Snack
Apple with Al-
mond or Peanut
Butter (p. 236)

Dinner
Veggie Burgers
with Green Salad
(p. 224)

DAY 21

Breakfast
Kale Juice
(p. 243) and a
hard-boiled egg

Lunch
Avocado Salad
(p. 195)

Snack
Cucumber Mint
Relish (p. 229)

Dinner
Arugula Salad
and Seared Tofu
with Melon
Dressing (p. 196)

DAY 22

Breakfast
Egg Spinach Wrap
with Beans and
Escarole (p. 205)

Lunch
Steamed Chicken
with Wilted Kale
and Raisins
(p. 220)

Snack
Tuscan Bean
Salad (p. 204)

Dinner
Stovetop Braised
Red Snapper
(p. 220) and
Wilted Spinach
(p. 235)

DAY 23

Breakfast
Apple with
Almond or Peanut
Butter (p. 236)

Lunch
Turkey Burger
(p. 222) and
Chopped Tomato
and Basil (p. 228)

Snack
Pea Mash
(p. 230)

Dinner
Roasted Turkey
and Steamed
Broccoli (p. 218)

DAY 24

Breakfast
Mango Smoothie
(p. 242)

Lunch
Puree of Broccoli
Soup (p. 190)

Snack
Mango Relish
(p. 202)

Dinner
Braised Salmon
and Steamed
Broccoli (p. 209)

DAY 25

Breakfast
Orange Salad
(p. 238)

Lunch
Roasted Turkey
and Steamed
Broccoli (p. 218)

Snack
Kiwi Dessert
(p. 242)

Dinner
French Chicken
and Braised Leek
(p. 210)

VEGETARIAN 25-DAY MEAL PLAN (NON-MEAT)

DAY 1	DAY 2	DAY 3	DAY 4	DAY 5
Breakfast	**Breakfast**	**Breakfast**	**Breakfast**	**Breakfast**
Pepper Onion Egg Wrap (p. 207)	Citrus Salad (p. 237)	Fresh Melon Compote (p. 237)	Mushroom Omelet Roll-Up (p. 206)	Tropical Fruit Salad (p. 240)
Lunch	**Lunch**	**Lunch**	**Lunch**	**Lunch**
String Beans with Sautéed Spinach (p. 234)	Puree of Broccoli Soup (p. 190)	Greek Salad with Tofu and Strawberry Dressing (p. 199)	Tofu Vegetable Soup (p. 191)	Roasted Root Vegetables (p. 232)
Snack	**Snack**	**Snack**	**Snack**	**Snack**
Tomato Gazpacho (p. 192)	Cucumber Mint Relish (p. 229)	Crudités with Dip (p. 229)	Choco Chestnut Pudding (p. 241)	Kiwi Dessert (p. 242)
Dinner	**Dinner**	**Dinner**	**Dinner**	**Dinner**
Grilled Tofu (p. 213) and Roasted Mushrooms (p. 232)	Roasted Eggplant Lasagna (p. 217)	Veggie Burgers with Escarole and Tomatoes (p. 223)	Roasted Eggplant and Tomatoes (p. 232)	Grilled Tofu with Kale and Sugar Snap Peas (p. 214)

DAY 6	DAY 7	DAY 8	DAY 9	DAY 10
Breakfast	**Breakfast**	**Breakfast**	**Breakfast**	**Breakfast**
Halved Grapefruit (p. 238)	Mushroom Omelet Roll-Up (p. 206)	Blueberry Smoothie (p. 240)	Kiwi Dessert (p. 242)	Kale Juice (p. 243) and a hard-boiled egg
Lunch	**Lunch**	**Lunch**	**Lunch**	**Lunch**
Beet Salad with Oranges (p. 197)	Vegetable Soup with White Beans (p. 194)	Puree of Broccoli Soup (p. 190)	Mexican Avocado Wrap (p. 215)	Spinach Kale Soup (p. 193)
Snack	**Snack**	**Snack**	**Snack**	**Snack**
Kefir Yogurt with Banana (p. 242)	Cucumber Mint Relish (p. 229)	Blueberry Applesauce (p. 236)	Tomato Gazpacho (p. 192)	Beet Salad with Oranges (p. 197)
Dinner	**Dinner**	**Dinner**	**Dinner**	**Dinner**
Veggie Stir Fry (p. 225) and Roasted Tomatoes (p. 231)	Ratatouille with Escarole Salad (p. 231)	Grilled Tofu (p. 213) and Roasted Vegetables (p. 232)	Veggie Burgers with Sesame Asparagus (p. 224)	Baked Sweet Potato (p. 226) with Wilted Spinach and Escarole (p. 235)

DAY 11

Breakfast
Papaya and
Blueberries
(p. 239)

Lunch
Greens with
Oranges and
Pumpkin Seeds
(p. 199)

Snack
Choco Chestnut
Pudding (p. 241)

Dinner
Grilled Tofu
(p. 213) and Pea
Mash (p. 230)

DAY 12

Breakfast
Citrus Salad
(p. 237)

Lunch
Chickpea Salad
(p. 197)

Snack
Blueberry Apple-
sauce (p. 236)

Dinner
Broccoli Rabe
with White Beans
and Peppers
(p. 227)

DAY 13

Breakfast
Egg Spinach
Wrap (p. 205)

Lunch
Roasted Root
Vegetables
(p. 232)

Snack
Beet Salad with
Oranges (p. 197)

Dinner
Veggie Stir Fry
Lasagna (p. 225)

DAY 14

Breakfast
Quinoa Porridge
with Apple
Compote
(p. 216)

Lunch
Tofu Vegetable
Soup (p. 191)

Snack
Fresh Pineapple
(p. 238)

Dinner
Steamed Veggie
Plate (p. 234)

DAY 15

Breakfast
Pear Apple Spice
(p. 239)

Lunch
Mexican Avocado
Wrap (p. 215)

Snack
Dried Mango
Slices (p. 237)

Dinner
Grilled Tofu and
Portobello Mush-
room Salad
(p. 200)

DAY 16

Breakfast
Strawberry
Smoothie
(p. 243)

Lunch
Greek Salad with
Tofu and Straw-
berry Dressing
(p. 199)

Snack
Tomato Gazpa-
cho (p. 192)

Dinner
Roasted Eggplant
Lasagna (p. 217)

DAY 17

Breakfast
Egg Spinach
Wrap with Diced
Tomatoes and
Chive (p. 206)

Lunch
Spinach Kale
Soup (p. 193)

Snack
Cucumber Mint
Relish (p. 229)

Dinner
Grilled Tofu with
Roasted White
Asparagus
(p. 214)

DAY 18

Breakfast
Tropical Fruit
Salad (p. 240)

Lunch
Avocado Salad
(p. 195)

Snack
Crudités with
Dip (p. 229)

Dinner
Veggie Burgers
with Escarole and
Tomatoes
(p. 223)

DAY 19

Breakfast
Kale Juice
(p. 243) and a
hard-boiled egg

Lunch
Vegetable Soup
with White Beans
(p. 194)

Snack
Sweet Potato
Corn Pudding
(p. 234)

Dinner
Ratatouille with
Escarole Salad
(p. 231)

DAY 20

Breakfast
Pineapple with
Blackberry Sauce
(p. 239)

Lunch
Grilled Portobello
Mushrooms and
Arugula (p. 230)

Snack
Kiwi Dessert
(p. 242)

Dinner
White Beans with
Peppers and Sugar
Snap Peas
(p. 226)

DAY 21	DAY 22	DAY 23	DAY 24	DAY 25
Breakfast	**Breakfast**	**Breakfast**	**Breakfast**	**Breakfast**
Kefir Yogurt with Banana (p. 242)	Mushroom Omelet Roll-Up (p. 206)	Blueberry Smoothie (p. 240)	Sweet Potato Silver Dollar Pancakes (p. 221)	Fresh Papaya (p. 238)
Lunch	**Lunch**	**Lunch**	**Lunch**	**Lunch**
Beet Salad with Oranges (p. 197)	Vegetable Soup with White Beans (p. 194)	Puree of Broccoli Soup (p. 190)	Veggie Stir Fry (p. 225)	Spinach Kale Soup (p. 193)
Snack	**Snack**	**Snack**	**Snack**	**Snack**
Lentil Salad (p. 202)	Fresh Pineapple (p. 238)	Kale Juice (p. 243)	Avocado Salad (p. 195)	Choco Blueberry Pudding (p. 241)
Dinner	**Dinner**	**Dinner**	**Dinner**	**Dinner**
Grilled Tofu over White Romaine Hearts (p. 214)	Ratatouille with Escarole Salad (p. 231)	Veggie Stir Fry (p. 225) and Roasted Tomatoes (p. 231)	Baked Sweet Potato (p. 226) with Wilted Spinach and Escarole (p. 235)	Roasted Eggplant Lasagna (p. 217)

Tracy's Performance Cleanse Menu: Days 26–30

During the last five days of your kick start, the Performance Cleanse will help you shed weight to show off your beautiful new muscular structure. The last thing I want to do in this 30-Day boot camp is have you do a "liquid cleanse" for weight loss. Even though this is a "cleanse," it allows you to eat and feel full while your digestive system functions on a regular basis and you lose weight, fight cancer and other diseases, and promote longevity. Think real food instead of powders or diluted lemon juice and maple syrup. You get a high concentration of nutrients in portions that are consumable, that fight aging and disease—and that taste great.

I am not interested in you having your dream body for a weekend. I want you to own it for life. Extreme-calorie-reduction "cleanses" that have you drinking nothing but lemon juice and pepper "work." Every diet book on the shelf "works." But they work short-term. When you cleanse for a quick outcome and then go back to your regular patterns, the yo-yoing can cause potentially life-threatening damage. Fasting leads to muscle breakdown and can rob you of very important nutrients, not to mention throwing your body's natural chemistry off.

The Method Cleanse uses real food, so you are still digesting and getting maximum energy. Every day you will enjoy seven different foods that include sweets, savories, soups, puddings, and purees. These are:

Sweet Purees

Blueberry Applesauce

Kiwi Dessert

Choco Chestnut Pudding

Savory Purees

Edamame and Carrot with Cayenne

Sweet Potato Corn Pudding

Soups

Tomato Gazpacho

Chicken Protein Soup or Tofu Vegetable Soup

You'll have about four ounces of each food, and you'll eat as you need and desire to, whether this means nibbling throughout the day, grazing on larger portions at regular mealtimes and snack times, or combining the foods into three larger meals per day. Consider this to be luxury-style eating, pampering your body with nutritious, delicious food choices, just like you would for a child you were nurturing. Eat until your body is satisfied.

Along with the seven food choices, you'll also be able to drink Kale Spinach Beet Juice and Kale Juice for energy, as a snack, or to replenish your body after a workout. We all know that sitting down and eating pounds of kale would give us a lion's share of vitamins and nutrients, yet the thought is less than desirable to most. The beauty here is that you get the powerhouse benefits of all the carotenoids, chlorophyll, trace minerals, enzymes, and phytochemicals because this plan breaks down quantities that in solid form you'd be unable to consume.

By the time you begin your Cleanse, your body has already begun to change. At this point, you should be craving your daily exercise routine, have lost a significant amount of weight, and be enjoying markedly increased energy levels. Now you'll really take advantage of the thirty days of boot camp, and ramp it up. Now you can see the finish line—and you know you're going to make it.

The Sample Cleanse Menus

We all have different cravings and styles of eating. Even though this is a cleanse, I want you to feel satisfied, so I've identified a few common eating types and created sample menus for each. Remember: These menus are just samples. As long as you eat the seven prescribed foods in a day, four ounces each, you are doing the Performance Cleanse correctly.

1. **The Nibbler.** Some of us don't care if we never sit down to a meal. A handful of this and that every now and again, and we're satisfied. We'd rather be nibbling all day than loading up at mealtimes.
2. **The Grazer.** Not quite a nibbler that subsists on snacking, not quite someone who needs a full breakfast, lunch, and dinner, grazers enjoy light meals throughout the day.
3. **The Three Square.** Even if they're giving up mashed potatoes and gravy for the time being, these eaters are happiest sitting down to three full meals daily with a range of tastes and textures.

Below, you'll find sample menus for nibblers, grazers, and those who enjoy their three square meals a day.

The Nibbler

Nibblers are constantly craving food, and are happiest when there's always something on hand to eat. This sample menu allows you two ounces of food (or a green juice) every hour.

7 a.m.
Blueberry Applesauce (p. 236)

8 a.m.
Kale Spinach Beet Juice (p. 243)

9 a.m.

Kiwi Dessert (p. 242)

10 a.m.

Blueberry Applesauce (p. 236)

11 a.m.

Edamame and Carrot with Cayenne (p. 230)

12 p.m.

Kale Juice (p. 243)

Choco Chestnut Pudding (p. 241)

1 p.m.

Edamame and Carrot with Cayenne (p. 230)

2 p.m.

Chicken Protein Soup or Tofu Vegetable Soup (pp. 190, 191)

3 p.m.

Sweet Potato Corn Pudding (p. 234)

4 p.m.

Tomato Gazpacho (p. 192)

5 p.m.

Kiwi Dessert (p. 242)

6 p.m.

Sweet Potato Corn Pudding (p. 234)

7 p.m.

Chicken Protein Soup or Tofu Vegetable Soup (pp. 190, 191)

8 p.m.

Tomato Gazpacho (p. 192)

Choco Chestnut Pudding (p. 241)

The Grazer

If you're a grazer, you prefer eating smaller meals throughout the day to sitting down to a full meal three times. This sample menu is based on the principle of eating four ounces of food every two hours.

7 a.m.

Kiwi Dessert (p. 242)

9 a.m.

Blueberry Applesauce (p. 236)

11 a.m.

Kale Spinach Beet Juice (p. 243)

1 p.m.

Edamame and Carrot with Cayenne (p. 230)

3 p.m.

Tomato Gazpacho (p. 192)

5 p.m.

Sweet Potato Corn Pudding (p. 234)

Kale Juice (p. 243)

7 p.m.

Chicken Protein Soup or Tofu Vegetable Soup (pp. 190, 191)

9 p.m.

Choco Chestnut Pudding (p. 241)

Three Squares a Day

Some of us don't like to constantly snack: Even when we're trying to lose weight, we still want to sit at the table with everybody else. This menu allows you to enjoy full meals with soup and dessert, and still support all the fantastic work you've done throughout the kick start.

Breakfast

Blueberry Applesauce (p. 236)
Sweet Potato Corn Pudding (p. 234)

Snack

Kale Spinach Beet Juice (p. 243)

Lunch

Tomato Gazpacho (p. 192)
Edamame and Carrot with Cayenne (p. 230)
Kiwi Dessert (p. 242)

Snack

Kale Juice (p. 243)

Dinner

Chicken Protein Soup or Tofu Vegetable Soup (pp. 190, 191)
Choco Chestnut Pudding (p. 241)

9

TA Method Menu Recipes

Lifestyle Menus and Performance Cleanse

Soups

CARROT GINGER SOUP

2 cups low-sodium vegetable stock, plus more on reserve
1½ cups peeled and chopped carrots
2 tablespoons chopped fresh ginger
¼ cup peeled and chopped Spanish onion
¼ cup peeled and chopped sweet potatoes
⅛ cup chopped celery
4 sprigs parsley, washed thoroughly
Fresh cracked pepper

Pour two cups of the stock into a heavy saucepan, then add the rest of the ingredients. Bring the soup to a boil and then reduce the heat, simmering until the vegetables are soft. Then puree the cooked mixture in a food processor. Add additional stock to correct the consistency.

Add freshly ground pepper and serve.

PORTION SIZE: 8 OUNCES

CHICKEN PROTEIN SOUP

½ cup peeled and chopped carrots

½ cup chopped celery

2 ounces boneless chicken breast, cubed, or 2 ounces Tofu, cubed

2 cups low-sodium chicken broth, or 2 cups low-sodium vegetable broth

½ cup chopped broccoli spears

2 tablespoons chopped parsley

Fresh cracked pepper

Simmer the carrots, celery, and chicken or tofu in the stock gently for 20 minutes, then add the chopped broccoli and cook for an additional 10 minutes. Add the parsley, season with pepper, and serve.

PORTION SIZE: 8 OUNCES

PUREE OF BROCCOLI SOUP

½ cup chopped celery

½ cup chopped onion

½ cup peeled and chopped sweet potatoes

1¼ to 1½ cups low-sodium broth (chicken or vegetable), divided

1 cup chopped broccoli

4 sprigs parsley

Fresh cracked pepper

Cook the celery, onion, and sweet potatoes for 5 minutes over medium heat in ¾ cup of the broth. Add broccoli, parsley, and ½ cup of broth; simmer for 20 minutes, then remove from the heat. Use an immersion blender to puree the soup, or puree it in batches in a food processor or blender. Add extra stock if you'd like a thinner consistency. Season with fresh pepper.

PORTION SIZE: 8 OUNCES

TOFU VEGETABLE SOUP

½ cup peeled and chopped carrots

½ cup chopped celery

2 cups low-sodium vegetable broth (or chicken, if you prefer)

½ cup chopped broccoli spears

1 tablespoon chopped parsley

2 ounces tofu, cubed

Fresh cracked pepper

Simmer the carrots and celery in the broth gently for 20 minutes. Add the chopped broccoli and cook for an additional 10 minutes. Add the parsley and tofu, season with pepper, and serve.

PORTION SIZE: 8 OUNCES

TOFU VEGETABLE SOUP WITH KALE AND SWISS CHARD

½ cup peeled and chopped carrots

½ cup chopped celery

2 cups low-sodium vegetable broth (or chicken, if you prefer)

½ cup chopped broccoli spears

1 cup chopped Swiss chard

1 tablespoon chopped parsley

1 cup chopped kale

2 ounces tofu, cubed

Fresh cracked pepper

Simmer the carrots and celery in the broth gently for 20 minutes. Add the chopped broccoli, Swiss chard, and kale, and cook for an additional 10 minutes. Add the parsley and tofu, season with pepper and serve.

PORTION SIZE: 8 OUNCES

TOMATO GAZPACHO

¼ cup chopped mixed bell peppers

½ cup chopped English cucumber

¼ cup cored and chopped sweet apples

⅛ red onion, chopped

1½ cups chopped tomatoes

1 teaspoon chopped chives

2 teaspoons chopped cilantro

Pinch of paprika

Pinch of cayenne pepper

Pinch of black pepper

Puree the first four ingredients in a blender for a few seconds to a small dice, then add the remaining ingredients and pulse until combined. (You can drain off some of the liquid if the gazpacho is too watery.) Serve chilled.

PORTION SIZE: 8 OUNCES

TOMATO MINESTRONE SOUP

2 cups low-sodium vegetable broth, divided

¼ cup peeled and chopped Vidalia onion

⅛ cup chopped celery

½ cup peeled and diced sweet potatoes

1 cup drained and chopped canned plum tomatoes

2 tablespoons chopped basil

1 tablespoon chopped parsley

1 tablespoon chopped chives

1 cup steamed fresh spinach

1 cup chopped and steamed kale

Fresh cracked pepper

Cayenne pepper

In a saucepan, combine ¼ cup of the stock with the onion, celery, and sweet potatoes. Sweat the vegetables for 8 minutes over medium heat, stirring. The stock will reduce and the vegetables will start browning. Then add the tomatoes and the rest of the stock, simmering until the vegetables are all soft. Add the basil, parsley, chives, spinach, and kale, and simmer for another 5 minutes. Season with black pepper and a pinch of cayenne, and serve.

PORTION SIZE: 8 OUNCES

SPINACH KALE SOUP

1 cup thoroughly washed and chopped leeks
½ cup chopped scallions (both green and white parts)
2 cups low-sodium vegetable stock, divided
1 cup chopped kale
1 cup chopped fresh spinach
1 tablespoon chopped parsley
Fresh cracked pepper

In a saucepan, braise the leeks and scallions in ½ cup of the stock, then add the rest of the stock and the kale, and simmer for 10 minutes. Add the spinach, and simmer until all the vegetables are tender. Then add the parsley, season with fresh pepper, and serve.

PORTION SIZE: 8 OUNCES

TURKEY KALE SOUP

2 pounds boneless, skinless turkey breast
6 cloves garlic, minced
4 sprigs rosemary
4 sprigs thyme
2 teaspoons soy sauce

4 cups low-sodium vegetable or chicken broth, divided

½ cup chopped Spanish onion

1 cup thoroughly washed and chopped leeks

½ cup chopped asparagus tips

½ cup chopped celery

1 parsnip, peeled and chopped

2 cups chopped kale

1 bunch parsley, minced

Fresh cracked pepper

Rub the turkey with half the garlic, half the rosemary, half the thyme, half the parsley, and the soy sauce. Place the seasoned turkey in a covered roasting pan into a 375-degree oven. Add 1 cup of stock into the pan, and then roast about 1½ hours, or until internal temperature reaches 165 degrees. Meanwhile, in a soup pot, add onion, leeks, asparagus, celery, parsnip, remaining thyme, 1 cup of water, and remaining cups of the stock. Cook for 10 minutes over medium heat. Reduce the heat to a simmer and cook for 20 minutes more, until the vegetables are soft. Strain the broth.

Cool the cooked turkey for about an hour, then shred it with a fork and add it to the strained broth. Chop the kale, add it to the turkey-and-broth mixture, and simmer for an additional 30 minutes. Serve garnished with parsley, seasoning with fresh pepper.

PORTION SIZE: RECIPE MAKES 4 SERVINGS

VEGETABLE SOUP WITH WHITE BEANS

½ cup cannellini beans

½ cup chopped carrots

½ cup chopped celery

½ cup chopped onion

½ cup peeled and chopped sweet potatoes

12 ounces low-sodium vegetable broth
½ cup chopped broccoli
4 sprigs of parsley
Fresh cracked pepper

To cook beans from scratch: One cup of dried beans will yield 2 to 2½ cups of cooked beans. Soak the desired amount of beans overnight in cold water. Strain and wash thoroughly. In a saucepan, slowly bring the beans to a boil and then cook over medium heat, until soft, about 1–1½ hours. Strain and chill under cold running water. Strain to remove all water. Set aside. (Or use canned beans.)

In the meantime, cook the carrots, celery, onion, and sweet potatoes in 6 ounces of broth for 5 minutes on medium heat, stirring occasionally. Add the broccoli, parsley, and 4 ounces of chicken broth and simmer for 20 minutes, then remove from heat. Use immersion blender to puree soup or puree in batches in food processor. Use remaining broth to correct consistency.

PORTION SIZE: 4 OUNCES

Salads

AVOCADO SALAD

2 medium avocados, diced
¼ cup chopped tomatoes, ¼" dice
2 tablespoons chopped sweet peppers, ¼" dice
1 teaspoon minced red onion
1 teaspoon chopped cilantro
Juice of 2 limes
Fresh cracked pepper

Combine all the ingredients, season with pepper, and serve chilled.

PORTION SIZE: 4 OUNCES

ARUGULA SALAD AND SEARED TOFU WITH MELON DRESSING

Arugula Salad

2 cups baby arugula greens

1 cup chopped tomatoes, ½" dice

¼ cup cooked corn

¼ cup sun-dried cranberries

½ endive, shredded

Seared Tofu (optional)

4 ounces firm tofu

Olive oil spray

Melon Dressing

½ cup seeded and chopped watermelon

Sprig of mint

Toss all the salad ingredients in a bowl and set aside. If you're using tofu, warm a sauté pan and coat it with olive oil spray. Brown the tofu for 2 minutes on each side, using a spatula for handling. Meanwhile, puree the watermelon with the mint.

Plate the salad and drizzle with Melon Dressing. Add tofu if desired.

PORTION SIZE: RECIPE MAKES 1 SERVING

BALSAMIC CHICKEN SALAD

4 ounces boneless chicken breast

2 ounces baby string beans (you can also use asparagus or broccoli)

¼ cup roasted peppers, no oil (can be store bought)

¼ cup chopped tomatoes

2 ounces balsamic vinegar

2 ounces orange juice

1 ounce fresh basil, chopped

Grill the chicken for 3 minutes on each side over medium heat, remove from heat, and then slice. Steam the baby string beans until soft, plunging them into an ice-water bath immediately to stop the cooking and so the beans retain their fresh green color. Toss the vegetables with the chicken. Thoroughly whisk together the vinegar, orange juice, basil, and 2 ounces of water, drizzle over the salad, toss, and serve!

PORTION SIZE: RECIPE MAKES 1 SERVING

BEET SALAD WITH ORANGES

1 cup peeled and quartered red or golden beets

1 cup vegetable stock

1 orange, peeled and sliced

Fresh cracked pepper

1 tablespoon chopped basil

Simmer the beets slowly in the stock until tender, then remove them from the liquid and cool. Reduce the remaining liquid by three-quarters and cool.

Arrange the sliced oranges on a plate and top with the cooled, sliced beets. Drizzle with reduced beet juice and season with pepper. Top with fresh basil.

PORTION SIZE: 4 OUNCES

CHICKPEA SALAD

1 12-ounce bag chickpeas (also known as garbanzos)

1 tablespoon diced red onion

¼ red pepper, seeded and diced

½ cup cored and diced sweet apples

1 teaspoon Dijon mustard with seeds

2 teaspoons rice wine vinegar

1 teaspoon chopped parsley

Soak the chickpeas for up to 6 hours, changing the water every 2 hours. At the end of the soaking time, wash the peas thoroughly under cold running water. Cook the peas in a large pot with ample water for approximately 2 hours at a simmer. Rinse and cool the peas thoroughly. (Or use three cups of low-sodium organic canned chickpeas.)

Toss all the ingredients thoroughly. Serve chilled.

PORTION SIZE: 4 OUNCES

GREEK SALAD WITH ENDIVE
AND RED ONION

1 cup chopped romaine

1 cup chopped escarole

½ chopped plum tomatoes

¼ cup chopped red onion

½ Belgian endive, cored, washed, and sliced

½ cup blanched string beans (boil for 5 minutes and chill immediately)

½ cup low-salt feta cheese

¼ cup pitted Nicoise olives

¼ cup chopped cucumbers

Juice of 1 lemon

Juice of 1 orange

Toss all ingredients and serve.

PORTION SIZE: 4 OUNCES

GREEK SALAD WITH TOFU AND STRAWBERRY DRESSING

Dressing

¼ cup red wine vinegar

½ cup fresh strawberries, pureed to liquefy

Salad

½ cup chopped English cucumbers

½ cup chopped tomatoes

⅛ Bermuda red onion, sliced

1 cup washed and chopped escarole greens

1 hard-boiled egg, peeled and sliced

½ cup diced firm tofu

Fresh cracked pepper

Dried oregano

In a bowl, combine the vinegar, strawberries. In a separate bowl, combine the vegetables, egg, and tofu. Pour the dressing over the salad, season with pepper and oregano and serve cold.

PORTION SIZE: 8 OUNCES

GREENS WITH ORANGES AND PUMPKIN SEEDS

½ cup chopped and seeded watermelon

Sprig of mint

1 orange, peeled and sliced.

1 cup baby spinach

2 tablespoons toasted pumpkin seeds

Puree melon with mint until smooth. Arrange sliced oranges on a plate. Top with spinach and dressing. Sprinkle salad with pumpkin seeds.

PORTION SIZE: 1 CUP

GRILLED CHICKEN OVER FRESH SPINACH SALAD

4 ounces boneless chicken breast
2 cups packed fresh spinach, washed thoroughly
¼ cup shaved fennel
4 tablespoons Dijon mustard
2 tablespoons red wine vinegar
Fresh cracked pepper
¼ cup dried cranberries

Grill the chicken for 3 minutes on each side over medium heat and then slice. Toss the spinach with the chicken and fennel. In a separate bowl, whisk the mustard and vinegar with 2 tablespoons of water, and season with pepper. Pour over the salad and mix thoroughly. Plate the salad fixings and top with the cranberries.

PORTION SIZE: RECIPE MAKES 1 SERVING

GRILLED TOFU AND PORTOBELLO MUSHROOM SALAD

Olive oil spray
1 portobello mushroom, peeled with stem removed
Fresh cracked pepper
2 ounces firm tofu
1 teaspoon yacón syrup

Heat up the grill or a frying pan. Spray the mushrooms with olive oil. Season with the pepper, and using tongs, grill both sides for approximately 3 minutes. Remove from the heat and place in a bowl. Cover with plastic wrap. This will allow the heat remaining to be trapped and "steam" the mushrooms while the tofu cooks.

Place the tofu on a baking sheet and brush with the syrup. Preheat oven to broil. Grill the tofu until crispy. Serve immediately with the mushroom.

PORTION SIZE: RECIPE MAKES 1 SERVING

GRILLED TOFU OVER WHITE ROMAINE HEARTS

¼ cup orange juice

⅛ cup rice vinegar

2 teaspoons yacón or agave syrup, divided

Fresh cracked pepper

2 ounces firm tofu

2 cups white romaine hearts, white and green leaves, chopped

Blend orange juice, rice vinegar, 1 teaspoon of yacón or agave syrup, and pepper thoroughly and set aside.

Preheat oven to broil. Place the tofu on a baking sheet and brush with 1 teaspoon of yacón syrup. Grill the tofu until crispy. Serve over romaine hearts and sprinkle with dressing.

GRILLED SALMON SALAD WITH ENDIVE AND RED ONION

Salad

4 ounces boneless salmon fillet

½ endive, shredded

2 tablespoons finely diced Bermuda red onion

½ plum tomato, chopped

Dressing

2 tablespoons raspberry vinegar

½ small cucumber, pureed

1 teaspoon chopped cilantro
1 tablespoon Dijon mustard

Grill the salmon for approximately 3 minutes on each side and cool. Flake about 4 ounces into small pieces. Toss with the rest of the salad ingredients in a mixing bowl and set aside.

Blend all the dressing ingredients in a blender until smooth.

Plate the salad, drizzle with dressing, and serve cold.

PORTION SIZE: RECIPE MAKES 1 SERVING

LENTIL SALAD

1 cup dried lentils
½ cup celery, finely diced in a food processor
2 teaspoons chopped chives
1 cup baby spinach
¼ cup golden raisins
Fresh cracked pepper
2 tablespoons grated parmesan cheese

Pre-soak lentils for two hours, then cook in 4 cups of water until soft. Drain, chill under cold water and drain again.

Mix the celery and chives with the lentils. Season with cracked pepper. Toss with the spinach leaves and raisins. Plate and sprinkle with the parmesan.

PORTION SIZE: 4 OUNCES

MANGO RELISH

1 medium mango, chopped into ¼" dice
1 tablespoon finely chopped red onion

2 sprigs cilantro, chopped

⅛ cup chopped sweet peppers (any color but yellow), ¼" dice

Combine the ingredients and chill.

SHRIMP SALAD WITH SUGAR SNAP PEAS

Dressing

Juice of 2 lemons

2 tablespoons sherry wine vinegar

1 teaspoon chopped cilantro

Salad

4 ounces (21–25) poached shrimp, peeled and deveined

¼ cup sugar snap peas, deveined (eat raw)

¼ cup hearts of palm, chopped

¼ bell pepper, sliced

Fresh cracked pepper

Whisk all three dressing ingredients thoroughly. Toss the shrimp and vegetables with the dressing. Season with fresh cracked pepper. Chill and serve.

SPINACH SALAD WITH CHESTNUTS

Salad

¼ cup sliced English cucumber

½ cup chopped tomatoes

1 hard-boiled egg, peeled and chopped

¼ cup chestnuts packed in water (not oil)

⅛ Bermuda red onion, sliced

2 cups washed and chopped baby spinach

Dressing

¼ cup balsamic vinegar

1 tablespoon Dijon mustard

Mix the salad ingredients and set aside. Whisk together the vinegar and mustard with ½ cup water and toss with the salad.

PORTION SIZE: 8 OUNCES

TUSCAN BEAN SALAD

½ cup cooked garbanzo beans

½ cup cooked red beans

½ cup cooked cannellini beans

1 teaspoon Dijon mustard with seeds

2 teaspoons rice wine vinegar

1 teaspoon chopped parsley

1 tablespoon diced red onion

¼ cup seeded and diced mixed peppers

½ cup cored and chopped sweet apples

1 cup chopped escarole

To cook dry beans from scratch: Soak all beans for up to 6 hours, changing water every 2 hours. After soaking, wash under cold running water thoroughly. Cook in large pot, on low heat, with ample water until soft. Cool and rinse. (Or use canned beans, drained and rinsed.)

In a small bowl, whisk the mustard with the vinegar and parsley.

Thoroughly toss all ingredients, including dressing. Serve chilled.

PORTION SIZE: 4 OUNCES

Eggs

EGG SPINACH WRAP

½ cup chopped spinach

1 teaspoon chopped fresh herbs: chives, basil, or parsley

3 egg whites, beaten

Olive oil spray

Fresh cracked pepper

Cook the spinach in a sauté pan until wilted. Remove and drain.

Combine the herbs with the egg whites. Heat an omelet pan and coat it with olive oil spray. Add the eggs to the pan. Cook until opaque white; do not stir. Add the spinach and fold the omelet. Season with fresh pepper.

PORTION SIZE: RECIPE MAKES 1 SERVING

EGG SPINACH WRAP WITH BEANS AND ESCAROLE

¼ cup cooked garbanzo beans

Olive oil spray

½ cup escarole washed and chopped

½ cup spinach

1 teaspoon chopped herbs: chives, basil or parsley

3 egg whites, beaten

Fresh cracked pepper

To cook dry beans from scratch: Soak garbanzo beans for up to 6 hours, changing water every 2 hours. After soaking, wash under cold running water thoroughly. Cook in large pot on low heat with ample water until soft. Cool and rinse. (Or use low-sodium beans canned in water, drained and rinsed.)

Heat saucepan over medium heat. Spray with olive oil. Stir in the escarole and cook for 2 minutes. Add the spinach and cook until wilted. Remove and place on paper towels to remove moisture.

Combine herbs with egg whites. Heat omelet pan and spray with olive oil. Add eggs to pan. Cook until opaque white; do not stir. Add greens and beans and fold omelet; cook for an additional 30 seconds. Season with fresh pepper.

PORTION SIZE: RECIPE MAKES 1 SERVING

EGG SPINACH WRAP WITH DICED TOMATOES AND CHIVE

1 teaspoon chopped chives
3 egg whites, beaten
Olive oil spray
¼ cup diced tomatoes
Fresh cracked pepper

Combine chives with egg whites. Heat omelet pan and spray with olive oil. Add eggs to pan. Cook until opaque white; do not stir. Add tomatoes and fold omelet. Cook for an additional 30 seconds. Season with fresh pepper.

PORTION SIZE: RECIPE MAKES 1 SERVING

MUSHROOM OMELET ROLL-UP

Olive oil spray
1 cup mixed chopped mushrooms
¼ cup chopped spinach
1 teaspoon chopped chives
2 egg whites
Fresh cracked pepper

Spray the pan with olive oil. Add the mushrooms and cook for 2 minutes. Add the spinach and cook until wilted. Drain and place on a paper towel.

Combine the chives with the egg whites and whisk. Heat an omelet pan and coat with olive oil spray. Add the eggs to pan. Cook until opaque white; do not stir. Add the mushrooms and spinach; fold the omelet and cook for an additional 30 seconds. Season with fresh pepper.

PORTION SIZE: RECIPE MAKES 1 SERVING

PEPPER ONION EGG WRAP

Olive oil spray
⅛ cup finely diced onion
⅛ cup finely diced pepper
3 egg whites, beaten
1 teaspoon chopped fresh herbs: chives, basil, or parsley
Fresh cracked pepper

Heat an omelet pan and coat it with olive oil spray. Cook the diced onion and pepper until soft; set aside and let them cool. Combine the eggs with the vegetable mix and the herbs. Spray the pan again with olive oil and cook the egg mixture. When the omelet has turned opaque white, fold it and cook for an additional thirty seconds. Season with fresh pepper and serve.

PORTION SIZE: RECIPE MAKES 1 SERVING

POACHED SALMON OMELET

½ cup vegetable stock
1 clove garlic, peeled and sliced
2 shallots, peeled and sliced
1 lemon, halved
3 ounces salmon filet

Olive oil spray
3 egg whites, beaten

In a shallow saucepan, bring the vegetable stock to a boil with the garlic, shallots, and lemon. Reduce and simmer for another 10 minutes. Add the fish, cover and barely simmer for about 6 minutes, until the fish is opaque. Remove fish with a slotted spoon. Flake with your fingers when cool to touch.

Heat omelet pan and spray with olive oil. Add eggs and cook until opaque white; do not stir. Add salmon and fold omelet, then cook for an additional 30 seconds.

PORTION SIZE: RECIPE MAKES 1 SERVING

VEGGIE OMELET ROLL-UP

¼ cup chopped and steamed spinach
¼ zucchini, grated
1 green onion, chopped and steamed
4 mushrooms, chopped and steamed
2 tablespoons quinoa, red or white (found in the health food aisle)
2 egg whites

Blend all the veggies together to make a puree; set aside. In a pan, bring ¼ cup water to a boil, add 2 tablespoons quinoa, then reduce the temperature to simmer. Cook until soft, about 10 minutes. Remove from heat, drain and chill. Add the chilled quinoa to the veggie mix. Cook the egg whites in a 10-inch ungreased nonstick pan to make a thin pancake. Add the quinoa and vegetable mix and fold the egg wrap over the filling. This dish can be made the night before; it's perfect for busy mornings.

PORTION SIZE: RECIPE MAKES 1 SERVING

Entrées

BAKED CHICKEN WITH BROCCOLI

4 ounces chicken breast, sliced

2 tablespoons plus 2 teaspoons orange juice

2 tablespoons agave syrup

½ cup low-sodium vegetable or chicken stock

1 cup broccoli florets, cooked until soft and drained

¼ sweet red pepper, sliced into thin strips

Preheat the oven to 350 degrees. Marinate the chicken in the orange juice and agave syrup for 15 minutes, then bake for about 12 minutes in an ovenproof nonstick saucepan. Carefully place the pan on the stovetop and put the chicken on a plate. Add stock to the pan and reduce the liquid. Toss the chicken with the broccoli and pepper, add the gravy, and serve.

PORTION SIZE: RECIPE MAKES 1 SERVING

BRAISED SALMON AND STEAMED BROCCOLI

1 cup vegetable stock

1 cup chopped braising vegetables (celery, leeks, carrots, etc.)

1 4-ounce boneless salmon filet

2 sprigs thyme

Fresh cracked pepper

2 cups Steamed Broccoli (p. 233)

Put ½ cup of the stock and the vegetables in a braising pan; cook for 3 to 4 minutes over medium heat. Place the salmon filet on top of the vegetables. Add thyme and season with pepper. Cover with the top and braise the filet on low heat for 6 to 8 minutes. Make sure the stock does not evaporate—add more if required. Remove fish with a spatula and plate with steamed broccoli.

PORTION SIZE: RECIPE MAKES 1 SERVING

FILLET OF WHITE FISH WITH OLIVES AND THYME

2 cups vegetable stock

¼ cup green pitted olives, sliced or whole

Whole lemon, sliced

2 sprigs thyme

1 6-ounce white fish fillet (you can use sea bass, cod, halibut, etc.)

In a small saucepan, heat the stock with the olives, lemon slices, and thyme, until boiling. Reduce the heat to a simmer, add the fish, and poach for approximately 8 to 10 minutes or until the fillet begins to break apart. Using a slotted spoon, plate the fish with the olives.

PORTION SIZE: RECIPE MAKES 1 SERVING

FRENCH CHICKEN AND BRAISED LEEK

French Chicken

Olive oil spray

1 10-ounce chicken breast (Ask your butcher to French cut it for you, giving you a boneless half breast with part of the wing attached.)

2 shallots, peeled and chopped

1 carrot, peeled and chopped

1 sprig rosemary

½ cup chicken stock

Braised Leek

½ leek, washed thoroughly and sliced

1 cup vegetable stock

Fresh cracked pepper

1 tablespoon chopped parsley

French Chicken

Preheat oven to 375 degrees. Heat a large, oven-proof sauté pan coated with olive oil spray over high heat. Place the French-cut chicken skin side down. Reduce to medium heat. Add the shallots, carrot, and rosemary. Cook for 4 minutes. Place the pan into the oven and roast the chicken for 12 minutes. Carefully move the pan to the stovetop, placing it over medium heat. Plate the chicken. Deglaze the pan by adding the chicken stock and using a wooden spoon to loosen all the ingredients and browned bits from the pan. Reduce the liquid by half. Strain and spoon some of the sauce over the chicken.

Braised Leek

Leeks can have grit embedded in the stalks, so be sure to trim and wash them thoroughly. Nothing is worse than sand in a dish you can't wait to eat! Preheat the oven to 350 degrees. Slice the leek in half lengthwise and place it in a small baking dish with enough vegetable stock to cover it. Season with pepper and parsley. Put it in the oven and braise for approximately 30 minutes, until the leek is translucent and soft.

PORTION SIZE: RECIPE MAKES 1 SERVING

GRILLED CHICKEN WITH BROCCOLI AND ENDIVE

1 6-ounce boneless chicken breast

1 cup broccoli florets

½ head endive, sliced

¼ tomato, diced

2 teaspoons honey

2 teaspoons balsamic vinegar

Grill the chicken for 3 minutes on each side over medium heat. Remove from the heat. (A thermometer inserted in the breast should read 165 degrees.) Meanwhile, prepare an ice bath for blanching. Bring water to a boil in a medium-size pot and add the broccoli; boil just until tender. Chill immediately in the ice bath. Cut the chicken into strips and toss well with the broccoli and remaining ingredients.

PORTION SIZE: RECIPE MAKES 1 SERVING

GRILLED CHICKEN WITH MANGO AND SCALLION

1 6-ounce boneless chicken breast
2 teaspoons sherry wine vinegar
2 teaspoons honey
1 teaspoon chopped cilantro
Fresh cracked pepper
½ mango, peeled and diced
1 tablespoon sliced scallions
¼ tomato, diced

Grill the chicken for 3 minutes on each side over medium heat. Remove from the heat. (A meat thermometer inserted in the breast should read 165 degrees.) Make a dressing by whisking together a teaspoon of water with the vinegar, honey, cilantro, and pepper.

Cut the chicken into strips and toss well with the mango, scallions, tomato, and dressing.

PORTION SIZE: RECIPE MAKES 1 SERVING

GRILLED FLANK STEAK

1 4-ounce flank steak
2 tablespoons Dijon mustard
1 clove garlic, minced

2 sprigs parsley, chopped
Fresh cracked pepper

Score the steak on both sides with a sharp knife. This prevents it from curling during the cooking process. In a mixing bowl, combine the mustard, garlic, and parsley; season with the pepper. Add the steak and cover thoroughly. Marinate for 30 minutes.

Preheat the grill. Place the steak on the grill and cook over medium heat. Grill 5 to 7 minutes on each side for medium-rare, or longer if a more well-done steak is desired.

Remove the grilled steak to a cutting board and let it rest in a shallow bowl for 5 minutes. Slice thinly on the diagonal. Spoon over the meat any juices released when it was resting and serve.

PORTION SIZE: RECIPE MAKES 1 SERVING

GRILLED LAMB TENDERLOIN

Olive oil spray
1 4-ounce lamb tenderloin, sinew removed (from Australia or New Zealand)
Fresh cracked pepper

Heat sauté pan over high heat. Spray the pan with olive oil spray, reduce heat to medium. Carefully place the tenderloin in the pan. Using a tongs, turn the meat to brown it on all sides. While it's cooking, season it with pepper. It should take only 5 minutes to reach medium. Remove from pan. Allow to rest for 5 minutes before serving.

PORTION SIZE: RECIPE MAKES 1 SERVING

GRILLED TOFU

2 ounces firm tofu
1 teaspoon yacón syrup

Place the tofu on a baking sheet and brush with the syrup. Preheat oven to broil. Grill the tofu until crispy. Serve immediately.

PORTION SIZE: RECIPE MAKES 1 SERVING

GRILLED TOFU WITH KALE AND SUGAR SNAP PEAS

1 quart veggie stock
1 cup sugar snap peas
2 cups chopped kale
Olive oil spray
1 clove garlic, minced
Grilled Tofu (p. 213)

In a large pot, bring the stock to a boil. Add the sugar snap peas and cook for 2 minutes. Remove from the pot with a strainer, chill under cold running water, strain, and set aside. Add the kale to the pot and cook for 2 minutes. As with the peas, remove with a strainer, chill under cold running water, strain, and set aside. Do not discard stock.

Heat a skillet coated with olive oil spray and sauté the garlic, stirring for one minute. Add the cooked kale and peas. Stir and add a ¼ cup of the original stock. Plate and serve the Grilled Tofu on top.

PORTION SIZE: RECIPE MAKES 1 SERVING

GRILLED TOFU WITH ROASTED WHITE ASPARAGUS

1 cup of white asparagus
Olive oil spray
Fresh cracked pepper
Grilled Tofu (p. 213)

Preheat the oven to 350 degrees. Coat a baking sheet with olive oil spray and place the asparagus on it. Roast asparagus for 5 minutes. Add pepper to taste. Serve with Grilled Tofu.

PORTION SIZE: RECIPE MAKES 1 SERVING

MEXICAN AVOCADO WRAP

2 medium avocados, diced
1 ounce diced tomatoes
⅛ cup diced sweet peppers
1 teaspoon minced red onion
⅛ cup cooked black beans
1 teaspoon chopped cilantro
Fresh cracked pepper
2 leaves red leaf lettuce

Toss together the avocado, tomatoes, peppers, onion, beans, and cilantro; season with pepper and chill.

Place the lettuce leaves—washed and patted dry—on a carving board or plate. Fill each with ⅛ cup of the avocado salad and carefully fold the lettuce around the filling. Slice in half and serve immediately. (These should not be prewrapped and eaten later, as the lettuce will become soggy.)

PORTION SIZE: RECIPE MAKES 1 SERVING

ORANGE GLAZED SALMON

1 6-ounce salmon fillet, skin removed
Juice of 2 oranges
2 teaspoons yacón syrup
Olive oil spray

2 sprigs thyme, chopped
½ cup vegetable stock

Preheat the oven to 375 degrees. Marinate the salmon in the orange juice and syrup for 15 minutes. Warm an ovenproof sauté pan and coat it with olive oil spray. Sear the salmon and cook it over medium heat for 2 minutes. Add the thyme, place the pan in the oven, and roast for an additional 4 minutes. (Do not turn the salmon over.)

Plate the cooked salmon. Move the pan to the stove over low heat. Carefully and slowly, add the vegetable stock to the pan, reduce the liquid to a syrupy consistency, and drizzle over the salmon.

PORTION SIZE: RECIPE MAKES 1 SERVING

POACHED COD

½ cup vegetable stock
1 clove garlic, peeled and sliced
2 shallots, peeled and sliced
1 lemon, halved
1 6-ounce cod fillet (you may also use halibut, tilapia, sole, or sea bass)

In a shallow saucepan, bring the vegetable stock to a boil with the garlic, shallots, and lemon. Reduce heat and simmer for another 10 minutes. Add the fish, cover the pan, and barely simmer for about 6 minutes, until the fish is opaque.

PORTION SIZE: RECIPE MAKES 1 SERVING

QUINOA PORRIDGE WITH APPLE COMPOTE

½ cup quinoa
½ cup apple juice
½ cup orange juice

1 sweet apple (such as Gala or Fuji)
¼ cup blueberries

In a saucepan, slowly cook the quinoa with the juices, stirring occasionally. This should take about 10 to 12 minutes. Meanwhile, steam the apple. Peel the apple and blend it in a food processor. Add blueberries and puree lightly.

Serve porridge as soon as it is ready, topping it with the fruit compote.

PORTION SIZE: 4 OUNCES

ROASTED EGGPLANT LASAGNA

Olive oil spray
1 medium eggplant, cut crosswise into ¾" thick slices
Fresh cracked pepper
¼ cup vegetable stock
½ cup chopped red onion
½ cup sliced cremini mushrooms
1 jar spaghetti sauce (organic, NO sugar)
2 cups Wilted Spinach (p. 235)
½ cup part-skim ricotta cheese
4 ounces shredded non-fat mozzarella cheese
3 tablespoons grated parmesan cheese

Preheat oven to 350 degrees. Spray a baking sheet with olive oil, place eggplant slices on sheet, and season them with pepper; bake for 15 minutes. Remove from the oven and cool.

In a heavy duty skillet over medium heat, add stock and onion; cook for 3 minutes, stirring occasionally. Add mushrooms and cook for 4 more minutes, or until mushrooms are tender, stirring frequently. Remove from heat.

In a 11-by-7-inch baking dish, starting with ¼ cup of spaghetti sauce on the bottom, create layers, using the tomato sauce, eggplant, mushroom mixture, spinach, ricotta, and mozzarella. The topping should be tomato sauce sprinkled with the parmesan cheese. Cover with foil and bake about 30 to 40 minutes until heated through.

ROASTED TURKEY AND STEAMED BROCCOLI

1 8- to 12-ounce turkey breast
½ cup chopped carrots
¼ cup chopped celery
¼ cup chopped onion
2 bay leaves
Cayenne pepper
Fresh cracked pepper
2 cups chicken stock, divided
1½ cups Steamed Broccoli (p. 233)

Preheat the oven to 350 degrees. Place the turkey in a roasting pan on top of a bed of the chopped carrots, celery, onion, and bay leaves. Season with the cayenne and fresh cracked pepper. Pour half the stock into the pan. Roast until the internal temperature of the turkey reads 165 degrees, approximately 20 to 30 minutes. Remove from the oven and place the turkey on a carving board.

To make the "gravy," place the roasting pan on top of the stove over medium heat; add the remaining broth. Bring to a boil and loosen the vegetables from the roasting pan. Reduce the heat and simmer. Allow the liquid to reduce to a silky consistency. Strain.

Slice the turkey to your desired thickness, plate next to the steamed broccoli, and dress with "gravy."

SEARED PEPPERED TUNA WITH ARUGULA GREENS

Olive oil spray
1 4-ounce tuna steak (sushi grade)
Fresh cracked pepper
2 cups baby arugula greens
Low-sodium soy sauce
Rice vinegar

Coat a sauté pan with olive oil spray. Season the tuna liberally with the pepper. Place the tuna in the pan and sear for 20 seconds on all sides. When the tuna is cooked, remove to a carving board and slice into ¼" thick strips.

Arrange the greens on a plate and sprinkle with soy sauce and rice vinegar. Arrange the seared tuna over the arugula salad, and enjoy.

PORTION SIZE: RECIPE MAKES 1 SERVING

SEARED TILAPIA WITH LEMON AND MUSTARD

1 4- to 6-ounce tilapia fillet
1 tablespoon Dijon mustard
Juice of ½ lemon

Preheat the oven to 375 degrees. Heat an ovenproof nonstick sauté pan and sear one side of the fish until brown. One side only! Brush with mustard and lemon juice, then finish cooking the fish in the hot oven for 3 minutes. Remove carefully with a spatula and serve immediately.

PORTION SIZE: RECIPE MAKES 1 SERVING

STEAMED TURKEY OR CHICKEN BREAST WITH WILTED KALE AND RAISINS

½ cup chopped carrots

¼ cup chopped celery

1 bunch kale, chopped

2 sprigs parsley

6 whole black peppercorns

1 bay leaf

1½ cups low-sodium vegetable stock

1 6-ounce skinless turkey or chicken breast

½ cup golden raisins

In a large pot, cover the carrots, celery, kale, parsley, peppercorns, and bay leaf with stock. Lay the poultry over the vegetables and steam, covered, until a meat thermometer inserted into the poultry reads 165 degrees. Remove meat to a carving board and allow to rest. Return the pot to the stove, add the raisins, and stir. Cook for 5 minutes. Plate veggie mix and serve with the sliced poultry.

PORTION SIZE: RECIPE MAKES 1 SERVING

STOVETOP BRAISED RED SNAPPER

½ cup peeled and chopped carrots

¼ cup chopped celery

2 shallots, peeled and quartered

3 parsley sprigs

½ cup vegetable stock

1 6-ounce red snapper fillet, with skin

Place the carrots, celery, shallots, parsley, and stock in a small saucepan. Put the snapper on top. Cover and barely simmer for approximately 6 minutes, or until the fish is opaque. Remove carefully with a slotted spoon and serve immediately.

SWEET POTATO SILVER DOLLAR PANCAKES

1 egg white, whisked

2 tablespoons kefir (found in the health food aisle)

2 tablespoons flaxseeds

1 steamed sweet potato, mashed and cooled

Olive oil spray

3 tablespoons yacón syrup

Mix the egg white, kefir, and flaxseeds with the potato. Using a tablespoon, form the mixture into small pancakes. Coat a griddle with olive oil spray and set it over medium heat; place the pancakes on the griddle. Cook for approximately 1 minute on each side, flipping with a spatula. Pay attention when making these, as they can burn easily! They're best when served immediately. Serve with syrup.

TUNA FISH WITH ROASTED CAULIFLOWER
AND FENNEL

¼ fennel bulb, cored

1 cup cauliflower florets

Olive oil spray

3 ounces canned tuna in water, drained

Preheat oven to 350 degrees. Place vegetables in roasting pan and spray with olive oil. Roast the vegetables for 12 to 15 minutes. Remove and plate. Serve with the tuna.

TURKEY AVOCADO ROLL-UP

2 leaves red leaf lettuce
3 ounces thinly sliced Steamed Turkey (p. 220)
⅛ avocado, mashed into a puree
¼ cup finely chopped tomatoes
Pinch of chopped basil

Place the two lettuce leaves flat on a carving board and cover with a layer of turkey. Cover the turkey with the avocado puree and top with tomatoes and basil. Roll tightly, cut in half, and serve chilled.

PORTION SIZE: RECIPE MAKES 1 SERVING

TURKEY BURGER

¼ cup chopped onion
¼ cup chopped sweet peppers
¼ cup chopped celery
2 chives
4 sprigs parsley
2 sprigs cilantro
4 ounces ground organic turkey
Fresh cracked pepper
Olive oil spray

In a food processor, puree the vegetables and herbs to a fine, but not liquidy, consistency. Add the vegetables to the turkey in a bowl and mix well, seasoning with the pepper. Mold into two small burgers (they should be about 1 inch thick) and chill for about 20 minutes.

Preheat the oven to 350 degrees. Heat an ovenproof sauté pan and coat it with olive oil spray. Place the burgers in the pan and cook for approximately 3 minutes on each side, until crispy. Place the pan in the oven and finish cooking for another

5 to 8 minutes. The internal temperature of the burgers should be 165 degrees. Remove and serve.

PORTION SIZE: RECIPE MAKES 1 SERVING

VEGGIE BURGERS

¼ cup chopped onions
¼ cup chopped sweet peppers
¼ cup chopped celery
½ cup cooked chickpeas
2 chives
4 sprigs parsley
2 sprigs cilantro
Fresh cracked pepper
Olive oil spray

In a food processor, puree the onions, peppers, celery, chickpeas, and herbs, but do not liquify. Place puree in a mixing bowl, season with cracked pepper, and mold into 2 small burgers, about 1" thick. Chill for about 20 minutes.

Heat a sauté pan and spray with olive oil. Place the burgers in the pan and cook for approximately 2 minutes on both sides until crispy.

PORTION SIZE: RECIPE MAKES 1 SERVING

VEGGIE BURGERS WITH ESCAROLE AND TOMATO

Olive oil spray
1 clove garlic, chopped
2 cups chopped escarole
¼ cup vegetable stock
½ cup chopped tomatoes

Fresh cracked pepper
2 Veggie Burgers (p. 223)

Heat saucepan over medium heat. Spray with olive oil spray. Add garlic and sauté for 1 minute. Stir in the escarole and cook for 2 minutes. Add the stock and the tomatoes, and cook for another minute. Season with pepper and serve immediately with the Veggie Burgers.

PORTION SIZE: RECIPE MAKES 1 SERVING

VEGGIE BURGERS WITH GREEN SALAD

Romaine, red leaf, or green leaf lettuces
2 Veggie Burgers (p. 223)

Arrange your favorite greens on a plate. Top with Veggie Burgers and serve.

PORTION SIZE: RECIPE MAKES 1 SERVING

VEGGIE BURGERS WITH SESAME ASPARAGUS

3 ounces green asparagus
Olive oil spray
Fresh cracked pepper
½ teaspoon sesame seeds
2 Veggie Burgers (p. 223)

Preheat oven to 350 degrees. Remove the bottom 1½ inches of the asparagus stalk. Peel the remaining stalk. Place the asparagus on a baking sheet. Spray with olive oil. Season with pepper and sprinkle with sesame seeds and roast for 5 minutes.

Arrange on a plate with Veggie Burgers and serve.

PORTION SIZE: RECIPE MAKES 1 SERVING

VEGGIE STIR FRY

Olive oil spray
1 garlic clove, peeled and minced
½ cup peeled and sliced Vidalia onions
½ cup sliced mixed peppers
½ cup peeled and chopped carrots, ¼" slices
½ cup snow peas, veins removed
2 teaspoons fresh grated ginger
1 teaspoon minced lemongrass
½ cup vegetable stock
Fresh cracked pepper

Heat a large skillet on high heat. Coat the pan with olive oil spray and sauté the garlic, onions, peppers, carrots, and snow peas for 5 minutes, stirring constantly. Add the ginger, lemongrass, and stock. Cover and continue cooking for 3 minutes. Season with pepper and serve.

PORTION SIZE: RECIPE MAKES 1 SERVING

VEGGIE STIR FRY LASAGNA

Veggie Stir Fry (p. 225)
Roasted Tomatoes (p. 231)
¼ cup grated parmesan cheese

Preheat oven to 350 degrees. In a baking dish, create layers by alternating the Veggie Stir Fry and the Roasted Tomatoes until all have been used. The top layer should be the tomato sauce. Sprinkle with the parmesan cheese and bake for 20 minutes. Serve.

PORTION SIZE: 6 OUNCES

WHITE BEANS WITH PEPPERS AND SUGAR SNAP PEAS

½ cup cooked cannellini beans

1 cup sugar snap peas, veins removed

1 cup chopped mixed peppers, 1" dice

2 tablespoons chopped basil

½ teaspoon red pepper flakes

To cook beans from scratch: One cup of dried beans will yield 2 to 2½ cups of cooked beans. Soak the desired amount of beans overnight in cold water. Drain and wash thoroughly. In a saucepan, slowly bring the beans to a boil and then cook over medium heat, until soft, about 1 to 1½ hours. Drain and chill under cold running water. Drain to remove all water. Set aside. (Or use canned beans, drained and rinsed.)

Bring 1 pint of water to a boil. Add the sugar snap peas and cook for 2 minutes. Remove and chill under cold running water. Toss peas in mixing bowl with beans, peppers, basil, and red pepper flakes. Chill and serve.

PORTION SIZE: 4 OUNCES

Vegetables

BAKED SWEET POTATO

1 sweet potato, scrubbed and washed, with the peel still on

Preheat oven to 350 degrees. Wrap sweet potato in foil and place it on a baking sheet; bake approximately 40 minutes. To check that it is ready, use an oven mitt and gently squeeze the potato; it should be easy and soft to squeeze.

PORTION SIZE: 4 OUNCES

BRAISED LEEK

½ leek, washed thoroughly and sliced
1 cup vegetable stock
Fresh cracked pepper
1 tablespoon chopped parsley

Leeks can have grit embedded in the stalks, so be sure to trim and wash them thoroughly. Nothing is worse than sand in a dish you can't wait to eat!

Preheat the oven to 350 degrees. Slice the leek in half lengthwise and place it in a baking dish with enough vegetable stock to cover. Season with fresh pepper and chopped parsley. Braise for approximately 30 minutes, until the leek is translucent and soft.

PORTION SIZE: RECIPE MAKES 1 SERVING

BROCCOLI RABE WITH WHITE BEANS AND PEPPERS

1 cup white beans, cooked
2 cups broccoli rabe, stems removed
1 quart chicken or vegetable stock
Olive oil spray
1 cup chopped mixed peppers, 1" dice
2 cloves garlic, minced
2 tablespoons chopped basil
½ teaspoon red pepper flakes

To cook dried beans from scratch: Soak the beans overnight in cold water. Drain and wash thoroughly. In a saucepan, slowly bring the beans to boil in regular water. Remove again and drain. Chill and return to the pot; this time cook the beans, over medium heat, until soft. Drain and rinse under cold running water. Drain to remove all water. Set aside. (Or use canned beans, drained and rinsed.)

Blanch the broccoli rabe by bringing the stock to a boil. Add the broccoli and cook for 2 minutes. Remove with a tongs or hand strainer (retaining stock) and chill under cold running water. Strain.

Heat a skillet, spray with olive oil, and sauté the peppers and garlic, stirring. Add the cooked broccoli rabe and ¼ cup of the original stock. Add the beans, basil, and red pepper flakes. Mix thoroughly and serve.

PORTION SIZE: RECIPE MAKES 1 SERVING

CHOPPED TOMATO AND BASIL

1 cup chopped beefsteak tomatoes
2 tablespoons chopped basil
Fresh cracked pepper

Toss all ingredients and serve chilled.

PORTION SIZE: 4 OUNCES

CORN AND SWEET PEPPERS

2 ears corn
1 sweet red pepper
Olive oil spray
Fresh cracked pepper

Preheat the oven to 375 degrees. Slice the kernels of corn off the cob and slice the red pepper into strips. Place the vegetables in a roasting pan coated with olive oil spray. Season with fresh cracked pepper. Roast for approximately 5 to 10 minutes.

PORTION SIZE: RECIPE MAKES 1 SERVING

CRUDITÉS WITH DIP

Dip

2 tablespoons sherry wine vinegar

2 tablespoons honey

Juice of 1 lemon

2 basil leaves, chopped

Fresh cracked pepper

Crudités

¼ cup carrot sticks

¼ cup celery sticks

¼ cup jicama sticks

⅛ cup cherry tomatoes

⅛ cup julienned bell peppers

Whisk the vinegar, honey, lemon juice, basil, and pepper, and serve alongside the vegetables.

PORTION SIZE: RECIPE MAKES 1 SERVING

CUCUMBER MINT RELISH

1 English cucumber, finely chopped

½ cup shelled and steamed edamame (can be purchased shelled and frozen)

2 tablespoons coconut water

2 teaspoons chopped fresh mint

Toss all the ingredients together. This relish can be made a day ahead. Serve it with fish entrées or snacks.

PORTION SIZE: RECIPE MAKES 1 SERVING

EDAMAME AND CARROT WITH CAYENNE

¾ cup shelled edamame
1 carrot, chopped
Handful of raw spinach
Pinch of cayenne pepper

Steam the edamame and carrot. Blend the steamed vegetables with the raw spinach and cayenne pepper. Add water as needed to thin the mixture for blending.

PORTION SIZE: 8 OUNCES

GRILLED PORTOBELLO MUSHROOMS AND ARUGULA

2 portobello mushrooms, peeled and stems removed
Olive oil spray
Fresh cracked pepper
2 cups baby arugula
1 Meyer lemon

Preheat the grill. Spray the mushrooms with olive oil. Season with the pepper and, using a tongs, grill both sides for about 3 minutes each. Remove from the heat and place in a bowl. Cover with plastic wrap. This will allow the remaining heat to be trapped and "steam" the mushrooms.

Dress your plate with the greens and drizzle with squeezed lemon. Slice the mushrooms and serve with the greens. (You can also spoon some of the mushroom juice on your greens.)

PORTION SIZE: RECIPE MAKES 1 SERVING

PEA MASH

¾ cup edamame, spring peas, or snow peas
Fresh cracked pepper

Steam the soybeans or peas over stock or water until soft. Mash and season with pepper.

PORTION SIZE: RECIPE MAKES 1 SERVING

RATATOUILLE WITH ESCAROLE SALAD

¼ cup chopped Spanish onion, ½" dice

1 cup seeded and chopped red and green peppers, ½" dice

2 cloves garlic, minced

1 cup chopped zucchini, ½" dice

1 cup chopped eggplant, ½" dice

1 cup chopped tomatoes, ½" dice

4 tablespoons chopped basil

¼ teaspoon oregano

Fresh cracked pepper

1 cup escarole

Fresh lemon wedge, if desired

In a large skillet on high heat, sauté the onion and peppers with the garlic. After 2 minutes, reduce heat to medium. Add the zucchini and eggplant and stir in thoroughly; cook for 10 minutes. Add the tomatoes and herbs, season with the cracked pepper, and cook another 10 minutes. Serve alongside escarole dressed with a squeeze of lemon.

PORTION SIZE: RECIPE MAKES 1 SERVING

ROASTED TOMATOES

6 plum tomatoes

Fresh cracked pepper

6 tablespoons chopped basil

Preheat oven to 350 degrees. Cut the tomatoes in half and place on baking sheet, cut side up. Season with pepper and basil. Roast the tomatoes for 15 minutes. Remove from the oven, puree in a blender or food processor, and serve.

PORTION SIZE: RECIPE MAKES 1 SERVING

ROASTED ROOT VEGETABLES

Olive oil spray
½ cup chopped turnips, 1" chunks
½ cup chopped carrots, 1" chunks
½ cup chopped parsnips, 1" chunks
Fresh cracked pepper
1 tablespoon chopped parsley
Ground chili powder
Juice of 1 lemon
½ cup baby pearl or cipollini onions

Preheat the oven to 375 degrees. Coat a roasting pan with olive oil spray, add the turnips, carrots, and parsnips, and spray them with olive oil. Season them with fresh pepper, parsley, chili powder, and lemon juice, and stir. Roast for 10 minutes, and then add the onions and stir. Roast for 10 more minutes or until done.

PORTION SIZE: RECIPE MAKES 1 SERVING

ROASTED VEGETABLES (ASPARAGUS, BRUSSELS SPROUTS, MUSHROOMS, EGGPLANT, TOMATOES)

Vegetables of your choice, washed and trimmed as needed (cut Brussels
*   sprouts in half)*
1 lemon
Fresh cracked pepper

Preheat the oven to 350 degrees. Place the vegetables on a baking sheet coated with organic olive oil spray. Put in oven and roast for appropriate amount of time: asparagus, 5 minutes; mushrooms, 3 to 5 minutes; Brussels sprouts, 15 minutes; eggplant, 15 minutes; tomatoes, 5 minutes.

Remove from the oven and drizzle with lemon juice and season with fresh cracked pepper.

PORTION SIZE: 4 OUNCES

ROASTED TRIPLE CARROTS

1 tablespoon maple syrup
1 tablespoon honey
1 cup vegetable stock, divided
½ cup peeled and quartered white carrots
½ cup peeled and quartered red carrots
½ cup peeled and quartered purple carrots
Fresh cracked pepper

Preheat the oven to 375 degrees. In a heavy, ovenproof saucepan, combine the maple syrup and honey with ½ cup of the stock. Add the carrots and roast for 20 minutes. Place the saucepan on the stovetop and deglaze with the remaining stock. Season with fresh pepper.

PORTION SIZE: 6 OUNCES

STEAMED BROCCOLI

Use a steamer basket or double boiler to steam broccoli over available stock or water for approximately 5 minutes. Make sure the florets are all the same size so that the broccoli will cook at the same rate.

PORTION SIZE: RECIPE MAKES 1 SERVING

STEAMED VEGGIE PLATE

½ cup peeled and chopped sweet potatoes, 1" dice

3 baby carrots, peeled and sliced lengthwise

1 cup vegetable stock

½ cup broccoli florets, hard green stems removed

3 white asparagus stalks, peeled

2 cups fresh spinach, washed thoroughly

Fresh cracked pepper

Steam the sweet potatoes and carrots over the vegetable stock until tender. Remove to a warming plate. Add the broccoli and asparagus to the stock and cook until soft. Remove to the same warming plate. Then wilt the spinach in the steamer, add to the veggie plate, season with pepper, and serve.

PORTION SIZE: 8 OUNCES

STRING BEANS WITH SAUTÉED SPINACH

½ cup green string beans

½ cup yellow wax beans

½ cup vegetable broth

½ cup spinach

Fresh cracked pepper

In a covered pot, simmer the string beans and wax beans in the broth until soft. Add the spinach. Cook for 1 more minute, then season with pepper. Serve immediately.

PORTION SIZE: RECIPE MAKES 1 SERVING

SWEET POTATO CORN PUDDING

1 sweet potato, peeled and diced

1 ear white corn

Steam the sweet potato. Slice the fresh sweet corn off the cob. Combine the ingredients in a food processor and puree, adding water as needed until you have the right consistency.

PORTION SIZE: 4 OUNCES

WILTED SPINACH

Olive oil spray
1 clove garlic, chopped
¼ cup vegetable stock
4 cups spinach

Heat a saucepan over medium heat. Spray with olive oil. Add garlic and sauté for 1 minute. Add the stock and spinach and cook for 1 to 2 minutes. Serve immediately.

PORTION SIZE: 4 OUNCES

WILTED SPINACH AND ESCAROLE

Olive oil spray
1 clove garlic, chopped
¼ cup vegetable stock
2 cups chopped escarole
2 cups spinach

Heat saucepan over medium heat. Spray with olive oil. Add garlic and sauté for 1 minute. Add the stock and the escarole and cook for two minutes. Add the spinach and cook for 1 minute more. Serve immediately.

PORTION SIZE: 4 OUNCES

Fruit

APPLE WITH ALMOND OR PEANUT BUTTER

1 apple sliced (Gala or Fuji)
2 tablespoons organic natural peanut butter or almond butter

For a healthy, simple to make snack, serve the sliced sweet apple with organic natural nut butter.

PORTION SIZE: RECIPE MAKES 1 SERVING

BERRY COMPOTE

1 cup mixed fresh berries, washed and drained thoroughly (your choice of strawberries, raspberries, blueberries, blackberries)
1 tablespoon pomegranate seeds

Toss the ingredients together. This recipe may be made the day prior.

PORTION SIZE: 1 CUP

BLUEBERRY APPLESAUCE

1 medium-to-large apple, quartered, cored, and steamed
1 cup fresh blueberries

Blend the steamed apple in the food processor with the blueberries and enjoy.

PORTION SIZE: ½ CUP

BLUEBERRIES AND BLACKBERRIES

½ cup blackberries
½ cup blueberries

Juice of 1 orange

Toss the ingredients together. This recipe may be made the day prior.

PORTION SIZE: 1 CUP

CITRUS SALAD

2 oranges
2 grapefruits
Juice of 1 orange

Peel the fruit, then cut into segments by carefully slicing between the interior membranes, segment by segment. This can be done by holding the fruit carefully in one hand and cutting with the other. Toss the ingredients together. This may be made the day prior.

PORTION SIZE: 1 CUP

DRIED MANGO SLICES

These can be found in most grocery stores or high-end markets.

PORTION SIZE: 2 OUNCES

FRESH MELON COMPOTE

½ cup diced honeydew melon
½ cup diced casaba melon
½ cup watermelon, seeded and pureed
1 teaspoon chopped basil

Toss the ingredients together. This recipe may be made the day prior.

PORTION SIZE: 1 CUP

FRESH PAPAYA

1 papaya, chilled and sliced.

PORTION SIZE: RECIPE MAKES 1 SERVING

FRESH PINEAPPLE

Serve sliced, fresh pineapple for a refreshing snack.

PORTION SIZE: 1 CUP

HALVED GRAPEFRUIT

½ teaspoon honey
1 grapefruit, halved and chilled

Drizzle honey on the chilled fruit and serve.

PORTION SIZE: 1/2 GRAPEFRUIT

HONEYDEW GRAPE SALAD

½ cup diced honeydew melon
½ cup red seedless grapes, halved
2 leaves basil, chopped

Toss the ingredients together. This recipe may be made the day prior.

PORTION SIZE: RECIPE MAKES 1 SERVING

ORANGE SALAD

2 oranges, peeled with white membrane removed
Juice of 1 orange

1 tablespoon chopped basil

Section peeled oranges and slice. Toss orange pieces with the freshly squeezed juice and top with chopped basil. Chill and serve.

PORTION SIZE: 4 OUNCES

PAPAYA AND BLUEBERRIES

½ cup chopped papaya
½ cup blueberries

Simply toss the fruit and chill.

PORTION SIZE: RECIPE MAKES 1 SERVING

PEAR APPLE SPICE

2 pears (Bosc or red), halved and cored
2 sweet apples (Gaia or Fuji)
Pinch of nutmeg
Pinch of cinnamon

Steam pears and apples until soft. Peel fruit and blend it in a food processor, adding spices as it purees.

PORTION SIZE: 4 OUNCES

PINEAPPLE WITH BLACKBERRY SAUCE

1 cup sliced pineapple
1 cup fresh blackberries, pureed

Pour blackberry puree over individual servings of pineapple.

PORTION SIZE: 1 CUP

STRAWBERRY MINT SALAD

1 cup sliced strawberries

1 teaspoon chopped mint

1 teaspoon agave syrup

Toss the ingredients in a mixing bowl to macerate. This recipe may be made the day prior.

PORTION SIZE: RECIPE MAKES 1 SERVING

TROPICAL FRUIT SALAD

¼ cup diced honeydew melon

¼ cup diced pineapple

¼ cup chopped papaya

¼ cup sliced kiwi

2 mint leaves, chopped

Toss the ingredients together. This recipe may be made the day prior.

PORTION SIZE: RECIPE MAKES 1 SERVING

Sweets

BLUEBERRY SMOOTHIE

8 ounces plain kefir probiotic yogurt (no sugar)

½ cup blueberries

Blend for a delicious smoothie. Make and chill 1 to 2 hours in advance of serving.

PORTION SIZE: 4 OUNCES

CHOCO BLUEBERRY PUDDING

½ cup semisweet chocolate chips
1 cup blueberries
1 tablespoon unsweetened cocoa powder

Melt chocolate slowly in double boiler and remove from the heat.

Blend blueberries in processor using the pulse option. Do not mush!

Add the blueberries to the melted chocolate. Add cocoa powder and, with a rubber spatula, blend ingredients together. Correct consistency with about ½ cup of water. Don't be afraid of too much water. Pudding will thicken as it cools.

PORTION SIZE: RECIPE MAKES 1 SERVING

CHOCO CHESTNUT PUDDING

½ cup semisweet chocolate chips
2 tablespoons peeled and cooked chestnuts
1 tablespoon unsweetened cocoa powder
4 whole pitted dates (you may substitute prunes or dried
blueberries)
2 tablespoons unsweetened coconut flakes

Melt the chocolate chips slowly in a double boiler and set aside. Puree the rest of the ingredients. Add the melted chocolate and pulse until all the ingredients are combined. Add about ½ cup of water and check the consistency. It should be soupy. Don't worry—it will firm up as it cools.

PORTION SIZE: 4 OUNCES

KEFIR YOGURT

Kefir can be bought in the refrigerated section of any supermarket. Look for flavored options!!

PORTION SIZE: 4 OUNCES

KEFIR YOGURT WITH BANANA

¼ cup plain kefir probiotic yogurt (no sugar)
½ banana, sliced

Mix yogurt and sliced banana and serve.

PORTION SIZE: 4 OUNCES

KIWI DESSERT

4 kiwis, peeled
12 basil leaves
Juice of ½ orange

Puree and chill.

PORTION SIZE: 4 OUNCES

MANGO SMOOTHIE

8 ounces plain kefir probiotic yogurt (no sugar)
½ cup chopped mango

Blend and chill for a delicious smoothie. Chill 1 to 2 hours before serving.

PORTION SIZE: RECIPE MAKES 1 SERVING

STRAWBERRY SMOOTHIE

½ cup strawberries

2 teaspoons chopped mint

8 ounces plain kefir probiotic yogurt (no sugar)

Using a blender, puree the strawberries. Add the mint and kefir; blend to a drinkable consistency.

PORTION SIZE: 4 OUNCES

Juice

KALE JUICE

1 bunch kale, washed and chopped

1 apple, peeled and cored (use Fuji, Golden Delicious, etc.)

Juice thoroughly, chill, and enjoy!

Hint: Try pears instead of apples!

PORTION SIZE: 8 OUNCES

KALE SPINACH BEET JUICE

3 leaves red kale

1 cup raw spinach, washed thoroughly

1 red beet, peeled

Juice everything and serve chilled!

PORTION SIZE: 8 OUNCES

OUR "BLOODY MARY"

2 cups chopped tomatoes

2 tablespoons chopped celery

1 teaspoon horseradish

1 red bell pepper, seeded and chopped

1 teaspoon chopped cilantro

1 sweet apple, peeled, cored, and chopped

Pinch of fresh cracked pepper

Pinch of cayenne pepper

Puree all the ingredients in a blender and serve chilled.

PORTION SIZE: 8 OUNCES

10

Frequently Asked Questions

Troubleshooting and Need-to-Knows

What If I Don't Have Time to Do the Complete Workout?

This is absolutely not my ideal scenario. Really, cutting your workout time short goes against everything I believe in. I'm giving you the truth here: It takes at least an hour a day to do my workouts. Truly, I want an hour and a half a day. This is a boot camp, after all. After thirty days, you'll thank me!

If you put in the time, and you master the musculostructure work with the complete understanding of how to perform the cross-vectors of force, and you can do forty-five minutes of cardio, then your body will change at an even ratio. Your muscular structure will change as quickly as you lose fat, which means that your skin tone will be the last thing that perfects, but it will perfect at a rate that matches everything. That's the ideal scenario. So do your best to make this ideal scenario part of your life.

If you only have fifteen minutes, you need to do your cardio. If you have weight to lose, and skin tone issues, and surface fat, and you have a short amount of time, the cardio is always my choice. Most people will turn to the muscular structure work first, because it's what they consider doable. But cardio goes the longest way if you only have a little time. So get moving, and squeeze the best out of whatever window you have!

If you only have fifteen minutes but you're doing forty-five minutes of cardio regularly, select the Muscle Design Work that homes in on your problem area: underarm flab, abs, or legs.

If you have thirty minutes a day, then you can choose either the muscular structure or the cardio. Alternate the days.

If you have one hour a day, six days a week, make sure that you are doing your muscular structure every other day, with fifteen minutes of cardio. On the alternating days, do the full hour of cardio, or do forty-five minutes of cardio, with muscle work on one of your target areas—the arms, abs, or legs—tagged on.

Is Cheating Allowed?

I am all about a lifestyle approach that works for you. I want you to make the fitness routine an important part of your life, but I absolutely understand the need for splurging and enjoying. The 30-Day Method is a boot camp, though, so I ask that you stay as true to it as possible—but you needn't take a radical cold-turkey approach. It all depends on the lifestyle you're starting from. If you usually consume alcohol, carbs, and dairy, and you don't work out at all, then making drastic changes all at once probably won't work for you in the long term. I want you to scale down. Stay as true to the 30-Day Method as possible, but if you're going out to dinner with family or friends, and you have a couple of glasses of red wine, don't beat yourself up over it, but dial it down to one night a week.

Until you can do forty to forty-five minutes of cardio a day, dripping with sweat, you really can't eat what you want. After you've done the 30-Day Kick Start, if you've achieved your desired results, you'll still do your cardio, you'll still do your muscular structure work—but you'll be able to eat more liberally and use the menus as needed to keep yourself in check.

What If I Want to Substitute Foods on the Menus?

I don't want you to make substitutions. But if you feel you must because of an allergy or a strong taste preference, make it a simple swap. You may not add anything new to the menu, but you may double up on another item from your daily menu if you really need to.

What If I'm Not Seeing Results?

If you're not seeing results, the first thing you need to do is go back to chapter 4 and work on your visualization and your connection. Are you turning your phone off? Are you really scheduling your time? You need to learn to troubleshoot for yourself. Ask the hard questions and give the accurate answers.

Often, when I'm in a follow-up session with a client who can't believe she hasn't seen results, I say, "Tell me what you ate yesterday. Did you follow the menu?" The first answer is, "Yes, I followed the menu." When we go through it step-by-step, however, every time I'll hear, "But I had only five almonds." Or, "I had three gummy bears." And, "Oh, I had four bites of my son's pasta, but that was it." Then we look at their workout time. "Well, you know, the washer went off, and I had to just stop for one second there."

What often comes out of these meetings is that the routine became a stop-and-go activity, which is not effective if you're after results.

You have to learn to hold yourself accountable. If you really believe that you are being 100 percent focused, and you are following the menus to a T, then maybe you aren't being challenged enough by the physical activity. That's when you need to look at adding ankle weights or upping the amount of time that you're exercising. Maybe your capacity is greater than what I'm challenging you with. Always make certain that you're really being tested, because there is no easy fix. So if the sequences or the cardio seems effortless to you, if you're not showing symptoms of challenge, you're not going to change.

If you stay accountable, focus, and don't become complacent, the changes you see will be remarkable, and they will keep you coming back for more.

One Last Note from Me to You

Dear Reader,

You and I have something in common: We both want you to look and feel amazing. That's why I wrote this book—because I want to make sure you're taking full advantage of the power that exists within you. If you let me design the plans for your perfect body and you learn to perform consistently, you will have the figure of your dreams.

For eleven years, I have focused on researching one thing: What can we do to achieve perfection? For eleven years, I have been developing all the tools that you need. Do you want your body to reach perfection? You can have it. I've succeeded in helping countless women like Gwyneth achieve these results.

My mission in writing this book was to share the message that you can get the results you want; now I want you to make it your mission to take advantage of what I am offering. I created the Method out of my own need for a real solution. It works, period.

Each one of you has different genes, different temptations, and different needs. This 30-Day boot camp is the first step toward your personal fitness goals. This approach to perfection recognizes that most of us are metabolically healthy; our choices have gotten us to wherever we are. Now, by consciously making new choices, we can repair what was done and restructure our bodies to our desired form.

Something to Keep in Mind

When you reach day 30 of the program, remember: A 30-day boot camp is just that—a boot camp—not a way of life. The menus will always be there if you need them later, but as long as you keep doing your Muscle Design Work, as long as you're really performing your Cardio Complement, you won't be on the menus forever. If you have a special event coming up, you can use the Cleanse or the Lifestyle Menu to slim down quickly. But these are not a way of life.

My approach to moving and eating *is* a way of life, and this book is just the beginning. This program will get you started down the road to a life of physical fitness. This kick start is exactly that: the catalyst you need to get from here to there. Thirty days from now, you can't just go back to the way you were living and eating. But you can't stay at a boot camp forever. You can't be on a diet forever. What you can do forever, however, is your workouts. Your Muscle Design Work—keep going, keep upping your reps. Your Cardio Complement: Keep working the steps, keep building fresh playlists. And in both cases, you can always check out my new DVDs for expanded routines and moves.

But that is then. This is now. Now it's boot camp time. Now we have a very specific goal: to shock your system. To rev up your engines. To get you kick-started into a routine that will give you the body you have always dreamed of. These are not empty promises. This is not a "five minutes a day" gimmick: This is the truth. This is hard work, but the kind of work that will get you where you want to be.

Give me thirty days. Follow my system. Let me train you. And together, we're going to wake up your whole body. You're literally going to be transformed. Your body will operate in a new way so that one day—maybe not today, maybe not tomorrow, but someday—you're going to spend an entire Sunday eating cupcakes, and as long as you've been doing the muscular structure work, and the cardio, and following my basic nutritional guidelines, you are not going to gain those pounds back. Ever. You're going to own your weight loss. You're going to own your recalibrated body.

You're going to own your life.

Do it for you.

Love,
Tracy

Acknowledgments

Tim Lambertson—You wouldn't be reading this if it weren't for him. He managed this project with so much heart as he does everything.

Rebecca Oliver—The most mindful agent on the planet.

Sandra Bark—A writer, a gypsy, a genius.

Bethany Karlyn—I can't bear to be photographed without her.

Miranda Penn Turin—She makes the word extraordinary seem lame. Her photography owns the truth from the most beautiful perspective.

Marc Mena—Some people just don't limit themselves to their recognized genius. What he can do with hair is every woman's fantasy but he also will never let you sport the wrong pair of shoes!

Grant James—Very few directors can direct with calm. When I film, the hours are long and physical. Grant is always thinking, creating, and manifesting around you without sucking your energy. He is young and incredibly gifted.

Karen Shapiro—I am petite and I know right away if I like something or not. I have listened to the wrong people in fashion before and always regretted it. Karen is on my wavelength and she watches my body language. She accentuates you with fashion not the other way around.

Diana Baroni—We all need that special someone who not only makes a dream a reality but actually cares about it. Diana got it from the start and is the kind of empowered woman I admire. To have her bring my first book to print is truly an honor.

Leila Porteous—Leila is like the amazing teacher that brings out your best without the tactic of fear. She nurtured the editing of my book in a mindful and protective way. With all of the projects I have going on, her guidance was a gift.

John Byrne—Well, when you give an incredible chef the strict rules that I have, to make something taste good you need a chef without an ego. John is so talented at making healthy satisfy the palate!

Grand Central—Thank you for believing in my talents, for giving me this wonderful platform to help people transform their health and happiness.

Index

Page numbers of illustrations appear in italics.

About the Author

Tracy Anderson is the creator of the Tracy Anderson Method, which has transformed the bodies of women across the world, including many well-known celebrities.

After more than a decade of research and testing, Tracy's mission is to capitalize on the hidden strength of the smaller muscle groups to give women a figure that is lean, long and feminine. With her exercise studios in Los Angeles and New York City, her line of DVDs, and now, this book, every woman can take advantage of Tracy's signature cardio and muscle work sequences.